# OMICRON
# &DELTA

Viruses Infection Long Hauler Symptoms
Diagnosis Patients and Physicians
Management Handbook

# OMICRON &DELTA

Viruses Infection Long Hauler Symptoms
Diagnosis Patients and Physicians
Management Handbook

## Dr. Frank Hamo

**To order additional copies of this book, contact:**
Xlibris
844-714-8691
www.Xlibris.com
Orders@Xlibris.com
839258

# CONTENTS

# *Section One Book Executive Summary*

## 1.0   Book Executive Summary

Emerging Very Highly Contiguous, Infectious and Transmissible Virus. The WHO classification as a VOC was based on epidemiological data indicating an increase in infections in South Africa in recent weeks that coincided with detection of Omicron variant.

Omicron has many concerning spike protein substitutions, some of which are known from other variants to be associated with reduced susceptibility to available monoclonal antibody therapeutics or reduced neutralization by convalescent and vaccine.

European Center for Disease Prevention and Control also classified this variant as a VOC due to concerns regarding immune escape and potentially increased transmissibility compared to the Delta variant.

This document discusses all emerging spikes and RBD mutation their effects on how virus will enter the human system and infect healthy cells.

Many people who have been sick with OMICRON/COVID-19, including some who had mild or no symptoms, reported dealing with additional symptoms long after their acute illness ended. The long-haul COVID-19 symptoms can range from fatigue or headaches to mental health issues or chronic pain, involving multi organs.

Some people have been suffering for more than a year with no answers, no treatment options, not even a forecast of what the future may hold.

Researcher and data collection on post COVID illness have identified number of illnesses involving multi organ symptoms, due to the fact when the virus enter the human system and the Cytokine storm triggered by the immune system to fight the virus can ravages human system randomly and causes multi system injury for healthy cells.

## 1.1 System can be affected by OMICRO/COVID 19 and can trigger long symptoms

A. Brain and Neurological System COVID Related Symptoms
B. Cardiovascular system COVID Related Symptoms
C. Respiratory System COVID Related Symptoms
D. Liver COVID Related Symptoms
E. Renal COVID Related Symptoms
F. Gastrointestinal system COVID Related Symptoms
G. Endocrine Systems COVID Related Symptoms

In this book will address each human organ and damaged tissues caused by previous COVID-19 infection by providing symptoms analysis and recommendation for imaging and screening.

**Note:** This book is intended to provide physicians with list of investigated post COVID sickness obtained from trusted scientific sources, symptoms management and treatment to be decided by health professionals. Symptom's treatment option is behind the scope of the book.

# Section Two OMICRON Spikes Mutation

## 2.0    Deep Dive into OMICRON Spikes Mutations

Since OMICRON virus had inherited spikes mutation from Delta and Beta viruses, therefore the following section intends to provide detailed information about OMICRON spike and RBD proteins mutation and amino acid proteins substitution that makes the virus very transmissible and infectious.

Items highlighted indicates that spike mutation has a property of high infection and ACE2 binding if infects the healthy human cells.

**Table one**: OMIRCRON Spikes and RBD

| RBD | Spikes |
|---|---|
| G339D | A67 |
| **S371L** | HV69-70 deletion |
| **S373P** | T95I, |
| **S375F** | G142D |
| **K417N** | VYY143-145 deletion |
| N440K | N211 deletion |
| G446S | L212I |
| **S477N** | ins214EPE |
| **T478K** | G339D |
| E484A | S371L |
| Q493R | **S373P** |
| G496S | **S375F** |
| Q498R | **K417N** |
| **N501Y** | N440K |
| | G446S |
| | **S477N** |
| | **T478K** |
| | E484A |
| | Q493R |
| | G496S |

## 2.1    Mutation Proteins

Table one and two lists OMICRON RBD and Spikes proteins mutation Against infection and severity

## 2.2    Proteins and Illnesses

Once the virus enters the human body it makes its way from upper to lower respiratory systems and infects health cells as results it depends on the virus entry points in association in what kind spike proteins facilitate cells entry and as results triggering illness from mild to sever

3

**Table two:** Isolating Proteins against Entry Points

| OMICRON Illness Managements | | | | |
|---|---|---|---|---|
| **Mild Illne Bronchus** | | **Sever Illnes Lungs** | | |
| S371L | Outer | D614G | Clear Entry | Epithelial |
| S373P | Proveins | K417N | Clear Entry | Epithelial |
| S375F | Clear ACE 2 | T478K | Interaction | RBD |
| S477N | Entries | N501Y | Interaction | PPI Interface |
| S371L | | N446K | Interaction | PPI Interface |
| S373P | | D796Y | Clear Entry | Epithelial |
| S375F | | G339D | Clear Entry | Endogenously |
| | | Q498R | Reduces ACE 2 Enzyme | |

**Table three:** Spikes Proteins Substitution

| | Proteins Substitutions | |
|---|---|---|
| **Spike** | **From** | **To** |
| S371L | Serine | Leucine |
| S373P | Serine | Proline |
| S375F | Serine | Phenylalanine |
| S477N | Serine | Asparagine |
| S371L | Serine | Leucine |
| S373P | Serine | Proline |
| S375F | Serine | Phenylalanine |
| G339D | Glycine | Aspartic acid |

| | | |
|---|---|---|
| G496S | Glycine | Serine |
| G446S | Glycine | Serine |
| **K417N** | Lysine | Asparagine |
| **T478K** | Threonine | Lysine |
| **D614G** | Aspartic acid | Glycine |
| Q493R | Glutamine | Arginine |
| **T478K** | Threonine | Lysine |
| Q493R | Glutamine | Arginine |
| T547K | Threonine | Lysine |

## 2.1  Substitution Proteins Impact

**S371L Leucine:** RBD, Infectious and Immune Escape

**S373P Proline:** Impact PCR Testing

**S375F Phenylalanine:** Strong infectivity and immune escape

**S477N Asparagine:** Increased AC2 binding

**S371L Leucine Spike:** Infectious and Immune Escape

**S375F Phenylalanine:** Strong infectivity

**K417N Asparagine:** Strong binding to AC2

**T478K Lysine:** Strong binding and infectivity

**D614G Glycine:** Strong binding and infectivity

**N501Y Tyrosine:** Strong transmission rates

**Table four:** Elements Molecular Structures

Table four below provides the reader reference of Mutations protein genomic molecular structures for the purpose of understanding the proteins molecular structures during virus mutation cycle.

Mutations Proteins Genomic Molecular Structures

| Name | Abbr | Labeled | Molecular Weight | Molecular Formula | Residue Formula | Residue VpKa1 (-H2O) | pKb2 | pKx3 | pI4 |
|---|---|---|---|---|---|---|---|---|---|
| Alanine | Ala | A | 89.1 | C3H7NO2 | C3H5NO | 71.08 | 2.34 | 9.69 | 6 |
| Arginine | Arg | R | 174.2 | C6H14N4O2 | C6H12N4O | 156.19 | 2.17 | 9.04 | 12.48 | 10.76 |
| Asparagine | Asn | N | 132.12 | C4H8N2O3 | C4H5N2O2 | 114.11 | 2.02 | 8.8 | | 5.41 |
| Aspartic acid | Asp | D | 133.11 | C4H7NO4 | C4H5NO3 | 115.09 | 1.88 | 9.6 | 3.65 | 2.77 |
| Cysteine | Cys | C | 121.16 | C3H7NO2S | C3H5NOS | 103.15 | 1.96 | 10.28 | 8.18 | 5.07 |
| Glutamic acid | Glu | E | 147.13 | C5H9NO4 | C5H7NO3 | 129.12 | 2.19 | 9.67 | 4.25 | 3.22 |
| Glutamine | Gln | Q | 146.15 | C5H10N2O3 | C5H8N2O2 | 128.13 | 2.17 | 9.13 | | 5.65 |
| Glycine | Gly | G | 75.07 | C2H5NO2 | C2H3NO | 57.05 | 2.34 | 9.6 | | 5.97 |
| Histidine | His | H | 155.16 | C6H9N3O2 | C6H7N3O | 137.14 | 1.82 | 9.17 | 6 | 7.59 |
| Hydroxyproline | Hyp | O | 131.13 | C5H9NO3 | C5H7NO2 | 113.11 | 1.82 | 9.65 | | – |
| Isoleucine | Ile | I | 131.18 | C6H13NO2 | C6H11NO | 113.16 | 2.36 | 9.6 | | 6.02 |
| Leucine | Leu | L | 131.18 | C6H13NO2 | C6H11NO | 113.16 | 2.36 | 9.6 | | 5.98 |
| Lysine | Lys | K | 146.19 | C6H14N2O2 | C6H12N2O | 128.18 | 2.18 | 8.95 | 10.53 | 9.74 |
| Methionine | Met | M | 149.21 | C5H11NO2S | C5H9NOS | 131.2 | 2.28 | 9.21 | | 5.74 |
| Phenylalanine | Phe | F | 165.19 | C9H11NO2 | C9H9NO | 147.18 | 1.83 | 9.13 | | 5.48 |
| Proline | Pro | P | 115.13 | C5H9NO2 | C5H7NO | 97.12 | 1.99 | 10.6 | | 6.3 |
| Pyroglutamatic | Glp | U | 139.11 | C5H7NO3 | C5H5NO2 | 121.09 | – | – | | 5.68 |
| Serine | Ser | S | 105.09 | C3H7NO3 | C3H5NO2 | 87.08 | 2.21 | 9.15 | | 5.68 |
| Threonine | Thr | T | 119.12 | C4H9NO3 | C4H7NO2 | 101.11 | 2.09 | 9.1 | | 5.6 |
| Tryptophan | Trp | W | 204.23 | C11H12N2O2 | C11H10N2O | 186.22 | 2.83 | 9.39 | | 5.89 |
| Tyrosine | Tyr | Y | 181.19 | C9H11NO3 | C9H9NO2 | 163.18 | 2.2 | 9.11 | 10.07 | 5.66 |
| Valine | Val | V | 117.15 | C5H11NO2 | C5H9NO | 99.13 | 2.32 | 9.62 | | 5.96 |

**Table five:** Isolating OMICRON Mutation Proteins against Infection and severity broken down between RBD and outer borders spike proteins

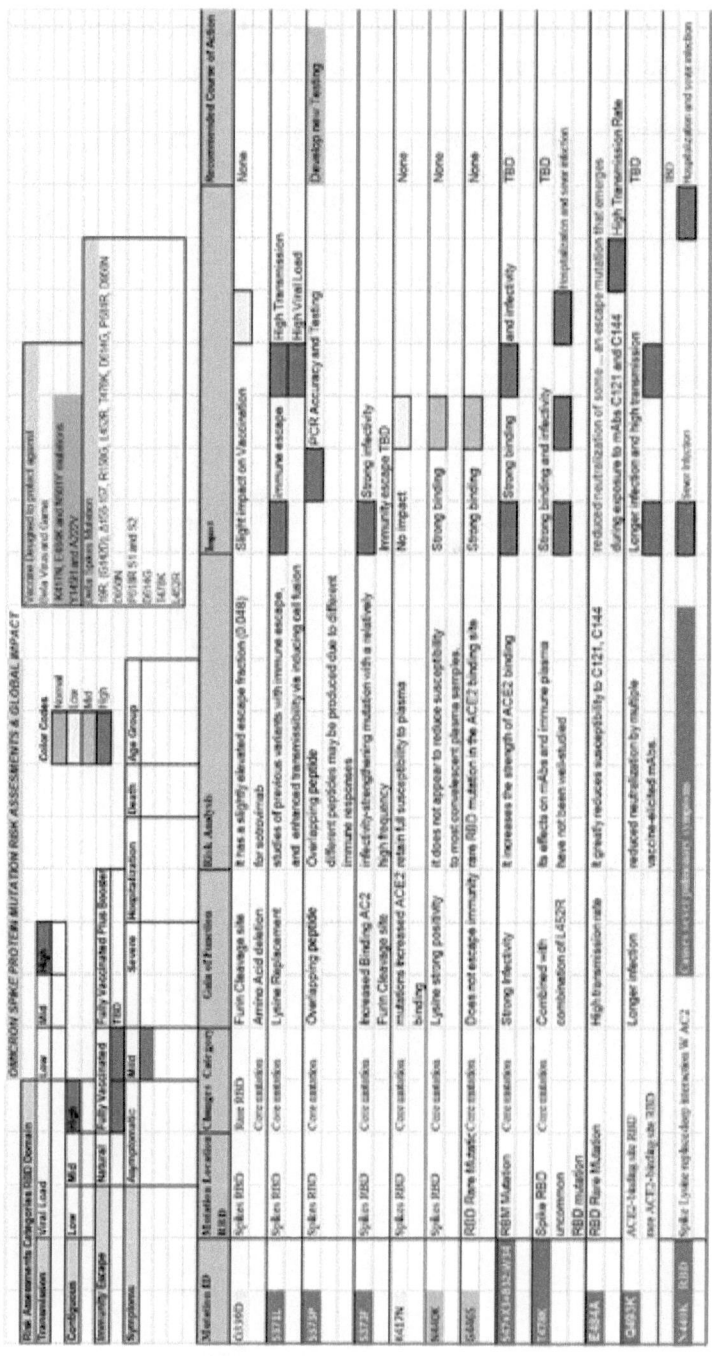

| Mutation ID | Mutation Location | Genome Changes | Codon Changes | Code of Function | Risk Analysis | Impact |
|---|---|---|---|---|---|---|

# Section Three Respiratory System

## 3.0 Upper Respiratory Tract Cellular Level

Upper respiratory tract includes the nose or nostrils, nasal cavity, mouth, throat (pharynx), and voice box (larynx). Virus enters through human respiratory epithelial layer which is composed of mostly ciliated cells with some secretory cells and basal cells. Secretory cells including serous, neuroendocrine and goblet cells,

**Figure one:** Nasal Mucosa Cells

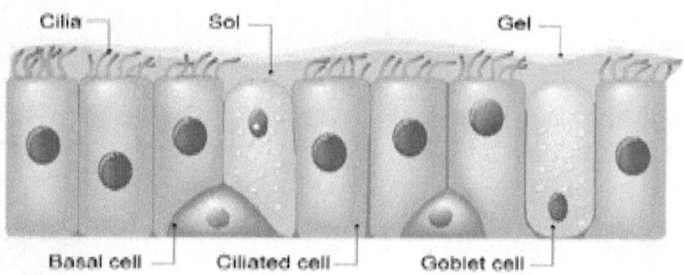

**Figure two:** Respiratory Epithelium

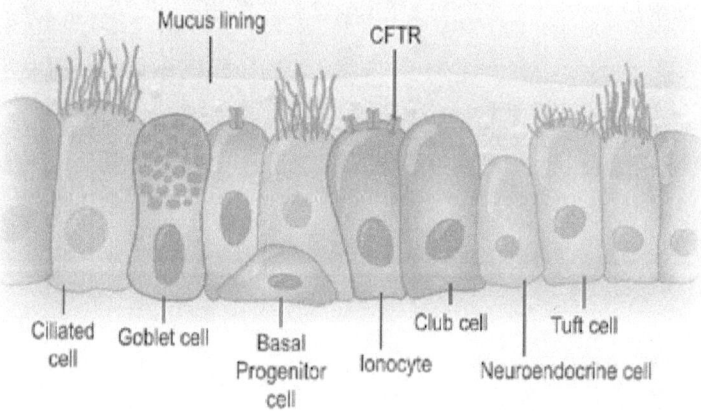

## 3.1  How Virus Enter Upper Respiratory Epithelial Layer

Virus enters through human respiratory epithelial layer which is composed of mostly ciliated cells with some secretory cells and basal cells. Secretory cells including serous, neuroendocrine and goblet cells. Ciliated cells facilitate the removal of foreign particles and debris via the mucociliary elevator. The viruses will infect the ciliated cells and replicate in upper respiratory tract, scientists relate the virus traps in upper respiratory tract and makes the virus highly transmissible.

## 3.2  OMICRON Infects the ACE2 Expressing Ciliated cells Upper Respiratory System

OMICRON infects the ACE2 expressing ciliated cells. SARS-CoV-2 replicates and infects neighboring cells. The ciliated cells initiate the innate immune response by secreting type I and type III interferons and other cytokines. The time from infection to initial release of virus is estimated to be about 6 hours. SARS-CoV-2 can dampen or delay the interferon and cytokine response compared with similar infections with influenza. The infected ciliated cells shed their cilia leading to impaired mucociliary clearance. In some areas, the epithelial barrier is severely damaged. The basal cells are spared from infection and can proliferate and restore the damaged epithelium.

## 3.3  Lower Respiratory Tract Explained

After the virus infects the upper respiratory system (Ciliated Cell), there is big chance giving all spikes mutation and their high infectious property to continue and invade the lower respiratory system including the alveolar epithelium is composed of type I and type II alveolar epithelial cells-type I alveoli epithelial cells enable gas exchange and type II alveolar epithelial cells secrete surfactant lipids and proteins helping to maintain the function and structure of the alveoli. Alveolar are responsible for gas exchange and any damage caused by infection will trigger sever sickness and in need of supplementary oxygen and mechanical ventilation.

**Figure three:** OMICRON Infection Difference between Lungs and Bronchus, Researcher Data for Illustration Purpose only

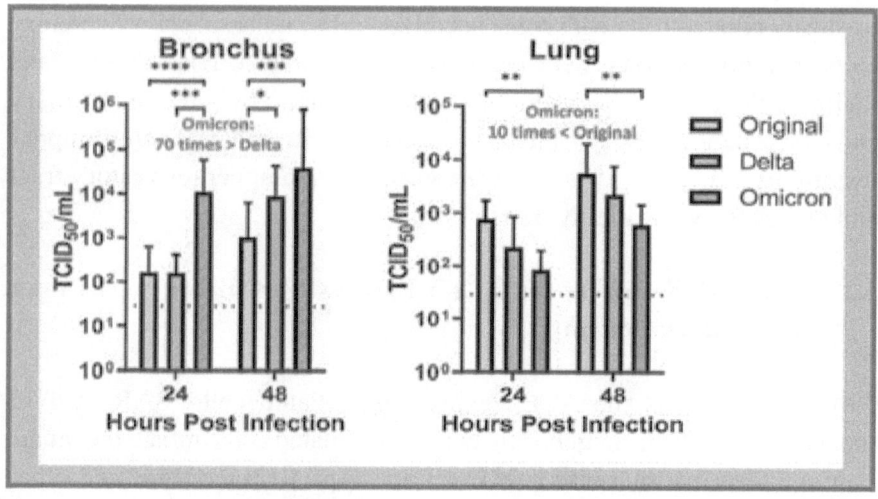

**Figure three shows the ratio of infections comparing bronchus against lungs**

**Figure four:** Human Respiratory Anatomy

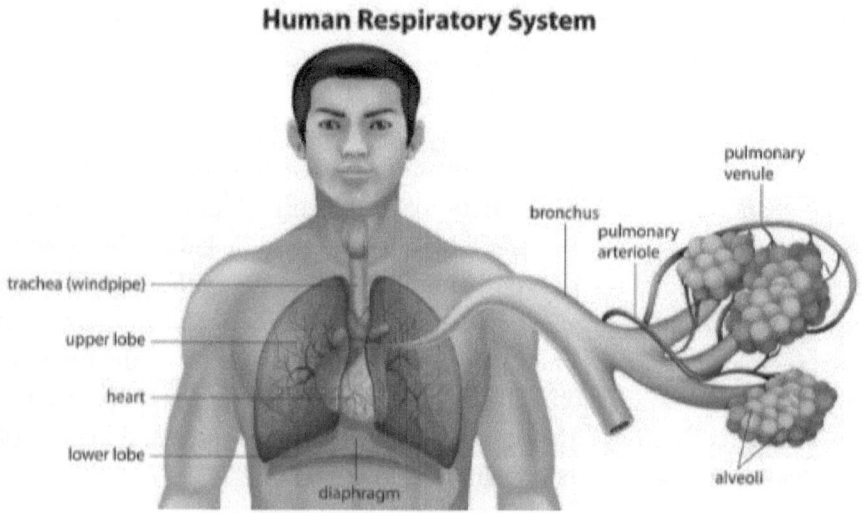

# Section Four OMICRON Transmissibility

## 4.0  Why OMICRON has High Transmissibility and Viral Loads

OMICRON outer border and RBD spikes having a property of being very strong AC2 binding near the cleavage area where no primer is needed that make viruses binding into the human healthy cells via AC2 much easier and faster, that factors make the virus incubation period much shorter than Previous BETA virus.

**Table six: *OMICRON Mutation Comparison between RBD and Spikes Proteins***

| Spike Protein Out border Mutations | RBD Mutations |
|---|---|
| S375P | N501Y |
| S371L | Y505H |
| S373P | K417N |
| N501Y | S471N |
| N440K | T478K |
| T478K | D614G |

| Delta Spike Proteins Mutations | | | | |
|---|---|---|---|---|
| T478K | D614G | P681R | D950N | L452R |

## 4.1  Mutations Comparison

Comparing mutation proteins between Delta and OMICRON as shown in table seven, Delta Mutations proteins: T478K, L452R and D614G. as noticed OMICRON has the same mutations protein: T478K, D614G proteins which they responsible for strong binding and severe infections. in addition, OMICRON carries N501Y proteins which makes the virus more transmissible.

## 4.2  OMICRON Higher Transmissibility Rates

Recent study had been noted those S proteins are in the outer border of the spike which makes it easier to bind to the first cells defense in the human upper airway and having higher AC2 expression comparing to lower respiratory system which has lower ACE2 expression, therefore virus replication is much high in the URT and trapped within URT and makes it very transmissible from one person to another.

When infected persons talk load, breath hard sheds viruses in the air and smaller droplets can stay in the air longer than large droplets that lands much faster, closed areas with unmasked gathering is a supper spreader area.

## 4.3 Why Children Get More Sicker Than Adults When Contracting OMICRON

During the current OMICRON pandemic, it has been observed that children at the age 0 to 4 years suffer more severe symptoms than adult patients. There has been speculation that this might be due to their ACE2 expression levels of the viral entry receptor, ACE2. Our results imply that there are no major differences in the epithelial expression of viral infection-associated genes between children and adults in the proximal airways.

During the current OMICRON pandemic, it has been observed that children suffer more severe symptoms than adult patients. Due to the age and their airways is much smaller than adults and any upper respiratory infection can causes implication of normal breathing therefor large number of children been admitted to the hospitals including the usage supplementary oxygen or mechanical ventilator.

# Section Five Sickness Managements

## 5.0 Infection & Sickness Managements

**Figure five: Respiratory System Detailed Diagram**

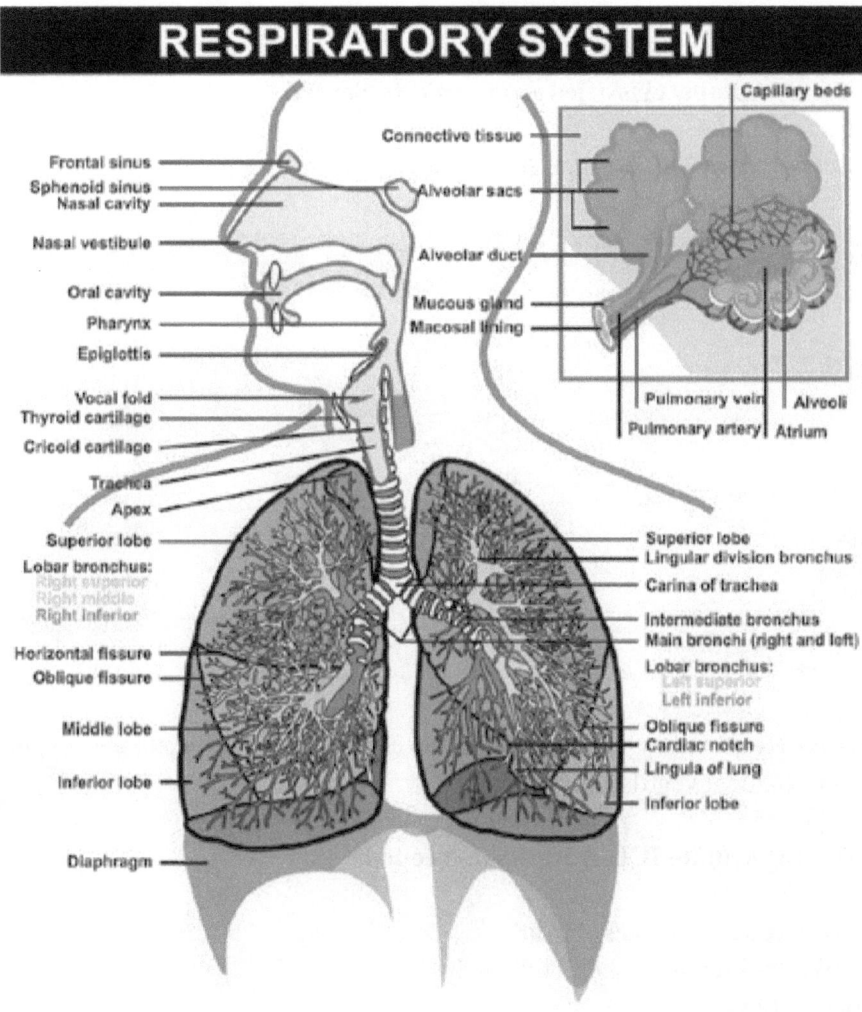

## 5.1 List of OMICRON Symptoms

During lungs infection the virus can escape from the lungs and enter the blood stream and invade multi-organ system tissues and triggers more symptoms

Here is a full list of 20 symptoms linked to Omicron top symptoms according to COVID reports and researcher data.

## 5.2 Symptoms classified from mild to Severe

**Table seven:** OMICRON/DELTA Defined Symptoms

| OMICRON Symptoms Diagnosis | | | | |
|---|---|---|---|---|
| Symptoms | Caused by OMICRON | | Caused by OMICRON Invades different Organs | |
| Headache | Temp for 3 days | Yes | Longer than 3 days | Neurological diagnoses is needed |
| Runny nose | Temp for 3 days | Yes | Longer than 3 days | Sinuses related |
| Fatigue | Temp for 5 days | Yes | | |
| Sneezing | Temp for 3 days | Yes | | |
| Sore throat | Temp for 5 days | Yes | | |
| Persistent cough | | | More than 5 days | Viruses start to infect LRT |
| Hoarse voice | Temp for 5 days | Yes | | |
| Chills or shivers | | | More than 5 days | Viruses start to infect LRT |
| Fever | | | More than 5 days | Viruses start to infect LRT |
| Dizzy | | | Cardiovascular system urgent diagnoses is needed | |
| Brain fog | | | Neurological diagnoses is needed | |
| Altered smell | | | Neurological diagnoses is needed olfactory | |
| Eye soreness | | | COVID 19 Related | |
| Unusual muscle pains | | | COVID 19 Related | |
| Skipped meals | | | Gastrointestinal diagnosis is needed | |
| Loss of smell | | | Neurological diagnoses is needed olfactory | |
| Chest pain | | | Delta Plumonary system infection immediate care is needed | |
| Swollen glands | | | COVID 19 Related | |
| Feeling down | | | COVID 19 Related | |
| Vomiting | | | Gastrointestinal diagnosis is needed | |
| Difficulty passing urine , Back pain | | | Renal System Delta related | |
| Note: Seems like OMICRON start invading different Organs: LRT, Bran, Renal System and Cardiovascular system | | | | |

**Lower Respiratory Systems Infection** can require supplementary oxygen or mechanical ventilation.

## 5.3 Immediate ICU Admission Needed

Severe cough Persistent Fever
Difficulty breathing shallow Breath
Blue tint to the skin
Rapid and difficulty breathing
Chest pain
Breathlessness, tight chest, or wheezing Muscle aches

**Chart one:** Admission Patient Survey Template for Patients to Complete

Patient Information Survey

Patient Name: _____ Age: _____
Patient Home Address: _____
Did you Receive Vaccine: Pfizer    Modena    J&J
When did you receive vaccine: _____
Did you get infected with COVID 19:    When: _____
Asymptomatic_____ Mild Symptoms_____ Sever Symptoms_____
Have you been hospitalized: _____
Supervised Medication Administered _____
Period Spent in hospital: _____
Time discharged from the hospital: _____
Please Check the Symptom That Applied to You

50 Most Common Long Hauler Symptoms

| Symptom | Yes | No | Explanation of Persistent Symptom |
|---|---|---|---|
| Fatigue | | | |
| Muscle or body aches | | | |
| Shortness of breath or difficulty breathing | | | |
| Difficulty concentrating or focusing | | | |
| Inability to exercise or be active | | | |
| Headache | | | |
| Difficulty sleeping | | | |
| Anxiety | | | |
| Memory problems | | | |
| Dizziness | | | |
| Persistent chest pain or pressure | | | |
| Cough | | | |
| Joint pain | | | |
| Heart palpitations | | | |
| Diarrhea | | | |
| Sore throat | | | |
| Night sweats | | | |
| Partial or complete loss of sense of smell | | | |
| Tachycardia | | | |
| Fever or chills | | | |
| Hair loss | | | |
| Blurry vision | | | |
| Congested or runny nose | | | |
| Sadness | | | |
| Neuropathy in feet and hands | | | |
| Reflux or heartburn | | | |
| Changing symptoms | | | |
| Partial or complete loss of sense of taste | | | |
| Phlegm in back of throat | | | |
| Abdominal pain | | | |
| Lower back pain | | | |
| Shortness of breath or exhaustion from bending over | | | |
| Nausea or vomiting | | | |
| Weight gain | | | |
| Clogged ears | | | |
| Dry eyes | | | |
| Calf cramps | | | |
| Tremors or shakiness | | | |
| Sleeping more than normal | | | |
| Upper back pain | | | |
| Flashes or flashes of light in vision | | | |
| Rash | | | |
| Constant thirst | | | |
| Nerve sensations | | | |
| Tinnitus or humming in ears | | | |
| Changed sense of taste | | | |
| Sharp or sudden chest pain | | | |
| Confusion | | | |
| Muscle twitching | | | |
| Feeling irritable | | | |

# *Section Six Limiting the Transmissions*

## 6.0 Managing OMICRON Transmissibility in Indoor and Outdoor Facilities

**6.1 Transmissibility:** due to the fact when a person gets infected with OMICRON the virus enters the upper respiratory system and infects the ciliated cells and replicate at very high rate, the reason is the upper respiratory system has higher **AC2** expression comparing to the lower respiratory system.

Therefore, the virus is trapped in the upper respiratory tract. When infected persons with symptoms speaks load, sneeze or caught since the viral load is very high due to high replication rates, he or she can shed very large amount of air born virus. Persons within less than 6 feet in closed area with no mask will diffidently contract the virus.

## 6.2 Limiting the Transmissions Rate in indoor facility

- a- Symptomatic persons should always wear certified mask
- b- Covering face when coughing or sneezing
- c- Noninfected person should wear certified mask and keep safety 6-foot distance
- d- Indoor gathering should be held with well-known family and vaccination status
- e- Indoor facility should have good ventilation system, prefers ultraviolet air system installed
- f- Frequent hands sanitization is recommended

## 6.3 Limiting the Transmissions Rate in outdoor facility

- a- Certified mask required in crowded street
- b- Be vigilant when someone passing you closer the 6-foot
- c- Small virus droplet can survive for few minutes before landed on the ground
- d- Hand's sanitizing

## 6.4 Managing unvaccinated Children from age 0 to 5 years

a- Parents should be fully vaccinated
b- Avoid any unknown visitor near child
c- Practice hands sanitization
d- Parents should wear mask near a child
e- Preferred to have a child sleep in different room
f- Avoid day care in the OMICRON time

# *Section Seven Long Haulers*

**7.0 System can be infected by:** DELTA virus and can trigger long symptoms

**Table eight:** OMICRON Mutation Proteins Responsible for Long Haulers and Organ Damages.

| OMECRON | | | | |
| --- | --- | --- | --- | --- |
| **Spike Protein Out border Mutations** | | | **RBD Mutations** | |
| S375P | | | N501Y | |
| S371L | | | Y505H | |
| S373P | | | K417N | |
| N501Y | | | S471N | |
| N440K | | | T478K | |
| T478K | | | D614G | |
| **Delta Spike Proteins Mutations** | | | | |
| T478K | D614G | P681R | D950N | L452R |

As shown in table eight OMICRON share some RBD and spikes protein as in DELTA, identified proteins: **T478K, and D614G**, these two proteins in delta virus are responsible for sever infection. In top of these two proteins OMICRON has more infectious proteins as: N440K, S371L and N401Y.

**7.1 Organs can be infected with OMICRON spikes proteins:**

A. Brain and Neurological System COVID Related Symptoms
B. Cardiovascular system COVID Related Symptoms
C. Respiratory System COVID Related Symptoms
D. Liver COVID Related Symptoms
E. Renal COVID Related Symptoms
F. Gastrointestinal system COVID Related Symptoms
G. Endocrine System COVID Related Symptoms

## 7.2 Long Haulers Symptoms

Do to the fact OMICRON inherited some of Delta Spikes and RBD proteins and these proteins can invade different organs and causes long sickness, the list below had identified 92 possible long hauler symptoms and all these information are obtained from trusted scientific sources all sources are identified within the content and some of these symptoms still under further investigation. All contents within are credited to the originator.

The list below is intended for physicians and patients for informational only
Physician recommendation is advised

## 7.3 List of Identified Symptoms from Trusted Sources

1- **Elevated Thyroid**: Some COVID-19 sufferers report having elevated thyroid levels as a long-lasting symptom of the virus

2- **Anemia:** Anemia is "a condition in which you lack enough healthy red blood cells to carry adequate oxygen to your body's tissues," says the Mayo Clinic. The most common type of anemia is associated with not getting enough iron. The condition makes you feel tired and weak. In some cases, it may even cause chest pain and dizziness, which are common long-lasting symptoms of COVID 19.

3- **Symptoms of herpes**: Epstein-Barr Virus (EBV), and trigeminal neuralgia are varied and may include fatigue, inflamed throat, fever, and facial pain. These are also common symptoms of COVID-19 and 38 sufferers who participated in the survey reported experiencing symptoms of these conditions after the virus was gone.

4- **GERD:** is acid reflux and it's commonly known to cause excessive salivation, or drooling. According to University of Florida Health, trauma, or infections in the throat, such as sinus infections or swollen adenoids, can cause GERD, which may lead to drooling. After COVID 19 recovery

5- **Personality changes**: Scientists are studying the rare but potentially *severe personality changes*: that COVID-19 may cause in patients. According to an article published in *Science News*, symptoms related to the brain are often overlooked as medical professional's focus on the physical aspects of the virus. However, depression, personality changes, and confusion are some long-lasting symptoms that some COVID-19 sufferers may experience.

6- **Thrush**: is small, white lesions inside your mouth caused by an imbalance of bacterial growth, more specifically an overgrowth of Candida, according to Cedars-Sinai. Some people are more prone to developing thrush, but it may also be common with COVID-19 survivors

7- **Hormone's imbalance**: Hormones are important because they regulate your appetite, mood, sexual function, and body temperature. According to Women in Balance Institute, a hormone imbalance may be caused by stress, an unhealthy lifestyle, or a buildup of toxins in the body. COVID-19 sufferers may experience this imbalance as the virus wreaks havoc on their respiratory system and as their immune system works hard to fight it off.

8- **Urinary tract infection** occurs when germs get into the urethra and begin to spread throughout the urinary tract, says to John Hopkins Medicine. One study published in Elsevier Public Health Emergency Collection "found a potentially dangerous overlap of classical urinary symptoms and the as yet not fully described symptoms of COVID-19." Urinary frequency and the virus may be related, which explains its potential cause of UTIs in patients.

9- **Kidney issues**: including protein in the urine, was a long-lasting symptom of COVID-19 for 47 survey participants. The specific ways the virus affects kidneys isn't known yet, but according to John Hopkins Medicine, it may invade kidney cells or the low levels of oxygen the virus causes may be what contribute to these long-lasting kidney problems.

10- **Dry scalp and dandruff**: can be uncomfortable and embarrassing. According to Cedars-Sinai, dandruff can be caused by changes in hormones, so it makes sense that it's related to the virus.

11- **low blood pressure**: such as genetics, your diet, or dehydration. According to the Mayo Clinic, low blood pressure is also related to infections and hormone fluctuations, which is why it may be a long-lasting symptom of COVID-19.

12- **COVID toes** are an emerging symptom of the virus that may not be as common as the other symptoms, such as cough or fever. COVID toes occur when the toes develop a rash or lesions. According to Dr. Humberto Choi, MD, from the Cleveland Clinic, rashes on the skin are common with viral infections such as COVID-19. The survey found that 59 participants had this strange side effect after being infected with coronavirus

13- **Eye Infection:** according to the University of Miami, it's possible that coronavirus could cause an eye infection, such as conjunctivitis, also known as pinkeye. The American Academy of Ophthalmology concludes that styes are caused by bacterial infections, which could explain the relationship to this eye condition and the virus.

14- **Foot pain**: can be caused by a few ailments, such as corns, plantar fasciitis, or Achilles' tendon injuries. "Covid toes" may contribute to this pain since some patients can have trouble walking or sleeping due to lesions on their toes. In most cases, this strange symptom goes away so, the foot pain should also subside.

15- **Goiter** is an "abnormal enlargement of the thyroid gland," according to the American Thyroid Association. While a goiter doesn't necessarily mean the thyroid isn't functioning correctly, it does indicate that there's a potential hormonal imbalance causing the thyroid gland to grow abnormally. 70 survey respondents dealt with a goiter after COVID-19, possibly due to the hormonal effects the virus has on the body.

16- **Cracked or dry lips** can occur in especially cold or hot weather or may be a sign of dehydration. When a virus like COVID-19 takes hold, dry lips may also occur because viruses are likely to cause dehydration. The American Academy of Dermatology suggests using lip balm, drinking plenty of fluids, and refraining from picking at the dry skin to get this symptom to go away.

17- **COVID-19** is a respiratory virus so it's no wonder those who contracted the illness feel a cold or **burning sensation in their lungs**. However, this symptom may last longer than the virus since 74 survey participants reported this feeling after coronavirus was gone. An article published in NBC News concludes that many COVID-19 sufferers felt this "slow burn" for a while, until it either worsened and was treated or went away completely.

18- **Bluish lips** according to the Centers for Diseases Control and Prevention (CDC), bluish lips or face is an emergency of COVID-19. When your lips turn blue, it's a sign your blood oxygen has dipped to extreme levels. The survey found that 77 participants claimed they experienced low blood oxygen after contracting coronavirus. One reason for this is that lung capacity may not have fully recovered from the respiratory virus.

19- **Arrhythmia** Mayo Clinic defines arrhythmia as a heart rhythm problem and explains it happens when "electrical impulses that coordinate your heartbeats don't work properly, causing your heart to beat too fast, too slow or irregularly." A study published in *Heart Rhythm* studied hospitalized coronavirus patients and found some of them suffered bradyarrhythmia or cardiac arrests. The study

concluded heart traumas and abnormalities like these are "likely the consequence of systemic illness and not solely the direct effects of COVID-19 infection.

20- **Jaw pain** in the survey, 80 participants reported jaw pain as a long-lasting symptom of COVID-19. According to the American Dental Association, jaw pain may be caused by bone problems, stress, infection, sinus issues, or tooth grinding. It's known that coronavirus causes aches and pains, so this jaw pain may be a lingering side effect of the body fighting off the virus.

21- **Painful scalp** COVID-19 sufferers, a painful scalp may be a side effect of the dandruff the virus may cause, or aches and pains associated with the illness. According to Kaiser Permanente, scalp pain or ailments may occur after recovering from a high fever, when dealing with a thyroid issue, or if you have poor nutrition

22- **Fizzing sensation:** according to an article published in *St. Peter's Health Partners*, a "tingling, burning, or 'fizzing' sensation" was reported from several COVID-19 patients. This sensation may be a side effect of other symptoms, such as aches and pains or fever.

23- **Back pain** According to the <u>National Institute of Neurological Disorders and Stroke</u>, back pain intensity can range "from a dull, constant ache to a sudden, sharp or shooting pain." Those recovering from illness may report this pain due to a decrease in movement over the past few days or due to the usual aches and pains of their sickness. 84 survey respondents claimed mid- back pain or pain at the base of their ribs after COVID-19. It's usually treated with muscle relaxants, gentle stretching, heat, or ice.

24- **Low temperature** After potentially experiencing a fever while fighting off COVID-19, sufferers may be surprised by the strange long-lasting symptom of a low body temperature once they've recovered. According to <u>Kaiser Permanente,</u> a low body temperature may occur with an infection or may be a sign of diabetes or a low thyroid level. A low temperature may also be the culprit for chills, since the body attempts to warm up with narrowed blood vessels

25- **Your veins circulate the blood around your** body and when you're too cold or hot, your blood vessels may constrict or widen. This may be due to having a fever, then low body temperature, or it may be a sign of dehydration. According to the <u>Mayo Clinic</u>, these bulging veins may be due to inactivity or damaged blood valves.

26- **Arthralgia** (joint pain) is a common symptom of coronavirus and a <u>study</u> published in the *Nature Public Health Emergency Collection* found that at least one patient in the 40 that were studied experienced joint pain. This joint ailment may linger in those who had the virus, causing hand or wrist pain to remain

27- **Costochondritis** <u>Mayo Clinic</u> defines costochondritis as "inflammation of the cartilage that connects a rib to the breastbone (sternum)." <u>Cedars-Sinai claims</u> that the risk for developing a chest wall infection like costochondritis is increased with respiratory trauma, such as pneumonia or bronchitis. Since COVID-19 is a respiratory illness, it's not surprising that 98 survey respondents who had the virus claimed costochondritis as a lingering symptom

28- **Spike in blood pressure** According to <u>Rush University</u>

Medical Center, a spike in blood pressure could be caused by a number of factors, such as stress, thyroid problems, or certain medications. A study published by the American College of Cardiology found a potential link between the virus and the renin- angiotensin aldosterone system, which is a "critical neurohormonal pathway that regulates blood pressure and fluid balance." This may explain the changes in blood pressure these patients experienced after coronavirus

29- **kidney problems** According to the National Kidney Foundation, acute kidney damage occurs in about 15% of COVID-19 patients, some of which never had kidney problems before. The survey found that 115 respondents have kidney pain after coronavirus, which may be a sign that the virus has caused kidney damage

30- **Brain pressures** the long-term extreme effects of COVID-19 remain a mystery, but the survey found that 119 people who had the virus suffered from brain pressure. A study published in the *Journal of the Brazilian Society of Tropical Medicine* found a potential link between COVID-19 and benign intracranial hypertension, a condition that causes pressure in the brain. These symptoms are usually temporary but can be serious if they get worse and are left untreated

31- **Swollen lymph nodes** According to the Cleveland Clinic, swollen lymph nodes are usually a sign that your body is fighting an infection. Your glands are working hard to flush out toxins and cells through lymph fluid. When your body fights a virus like COVID-19, lymph nodes may swell as all hands are on deck trying to get rid of the illness.

32- **Head Pressure** One of the common symptoms of COVID-19 is a headache but 128 survey participants reported feeling extreme pressure at the base of their head or occipital nerve after recovering from the virus. According to the American Association of Neurological Surgeons, pressure at the occipital nerve (the nerves that run through the scalp) may be caused by muscle tightness or pinched nerves. These nerves may experience pressure or pain during an infection or due to blood vessel inflammation.

33- **Rashes**: According to a study published in *JAMA*

*Dermatology*, the virus may be associated with a number of different skin rashes. The study found two different types of rashes that occurred in some patients infected with the coronavirus: petechial flexural eruption and digitate papulosquamous rashes. These skin conditions could occur at any time during and after infection and may contribute to the feeling of burning skin.

34- **Body, joint, and bone aches** are common with coronavirus and most other illnesses. According to one study, when the immune system is in overdrive, it causes an immune response that ramps up your white blood cells and causes them to produce glycoproteins called interleukins. These can cause joint pain, bone pain, and swelling

35- **Vessel irregularities** These feelings of hot blood rushing may be due to blood vessel irregularities caused by the virus or remnants of a fever. According to a study published in *Science Daily*, this sudden rise in temperature may be your immune system cranking up to continue killing off the virus. The study found that "elevated body temperature helps certain types of immune cells to work better.

36- **Chills without a fever** was a long-lasting COVID-19 symptom for 154 survey participants. It could be the body's way of continuing to regulate temperature and recover from a previous fever. According to Keck Medicine of USC, chills without a fever may also indicate your body is under stress and fighting a viral or bacterial infection or you're dealing with low blood sugar, which makes sense if you didn't eat much while you were sick.

37- **Neck pain** According to John Hopkins Medicine, your neck doesn't have much protection or support, so neck pain is common. Since the virus is known to cause muscle and joint pain, as well as body aches, your sensitive neck is more susceptible to this lingering symptom.

38- **Tongue pain and soreness** According to the University of Florida Health, tongue pain and soreness can be caused by several factors, such as infection, hypothyroidism, or a tumor in the pituitary gland. A study published in the *International Journal of Infectious Diseases* found that oral mucosal lesions may be associated with COVID-19 patients, which could explain this long-lasting virus symptom

39- **Heat intolerance** According to the CDC, one of the most common symptoms of COVID-19 is a fever. The body may need time after a fever has dissipated to recover and regulate its temperature. This may be why 165 survey respondents claim to have heat intolerance after being infected with COVID-19. As the immune system fights off the virus, it raises and lowers the body's temperature accordingly, which may cause this heat intolerance to linger.

40- **Swollen hands and feet** Those who contracted COVID-19 and experienced "COVID toes" or other skin- related symptoms may also be dealing with swollen hands and feet. According to the Mayo Clinic, this swelling is called edema and it could be linked to kidney or heart problems, both of which may be caused by coronavirus

41- **Dry skin** may be attributed to the rashes and cutaneous manifestations that some people develop on their skin due to the virus. However, according to the American Skin Association,

dry skin may also be attributed to a decline in fluid intake, which can happen when you're sick. It may also be a telling sign of a thyroid problem or hormonal imbalance

42- **According to A&D Medical**, "High blood pressure is not a documented symptom of COVID-19, but it can exacerbate the symptoms of the virus." The 181 survey respondents who report experiencing high blood pressure after having COVID-19 likely already suffered from this condition but fighting the virus may have made it worse.

43- **Living with a dry cough and sore throat** According to the World Health Organization (WHO), COVID-19 symptoms generally include a dry cough and sore throat. Living with a dry cough and sore throat throughout the course of the virus may cause this dry throat to remain for a while, even after testing negative for COVID-19.

44- **Post-nasal drip** is when mucus drips down the back of your throat and it's common after you've had a stuffy or runny nose. After dealing with allergy or sinus issues or infections, post-nasal drip can linger for a while. If one's body produced extra mucous and fluids to fight off the virus, this mucus may continue to drip. According to *Harvard Health Publishing*, you can treat post-nasal drip by staying hydrated, taking a nasal decongestant, or inhaling steam, such as from a hot shower.

45- **Weight Lost** COVID-19 survivors who had severe cases are likely to experience extreme weight loss. According to an article posted by Northeast Ohio Medical University, it's common for patients who survive severe infections or illnesses to lose weight. When sufferers are placed on ventilators or hospitalized for long periods of time, their bodies don't obtain the proper nutrition or muscle-building exercise. The body is also under stress fighting off the virus, which can cause this weight loss to occur. COVID-19 survivors who had severe cases are likely to experience extreme weight loss. According to an article posted by Northeast Ohio Medical University, it's common for patients who survive severe infections or illnesses to lose weight. When sufferers are placed on ventilators or hospitalized for long periods of time, their bodies don't obtain

the proper nutrition or muscle-building exercise. The body is also under stress fighting off the virus, which can cause this weight loss to occur.

46- **Feel irritable or angry**. According to *Med Page Today*, it's not uncommon for patients recovering from COVID-19 to feel irritable or angry. The virus may have mental health effects that make it hard for those who have recovered to go back to work or their daily routine without mood swings. Patients who were hospitalized may experience irritation and symptoms like post-traumatic stress disorder (PTSD) after being released.

47- **Muscle twitches** According to the University of Florida Health, muscle twitches may be caused by stress, lack of nutrients, or lack of sleep. Coronavirus is known to make its sufferers tired and their bodies stressed from fighting the virus, so this may explain muscle twitching. In some cases, it may be a sign of muscle damage or nervous system disorders.

48- **Mild confusion or "brain fog"** is a common symptom of coronavirus and most colds, flues, and viruses. According to an article published in *Science Magazine*, this confusion may occur because the body's systems are focused on fighting the illness, not giving enough focus, blood, or alertness to the brain.

49- **Lungs Pressure:** According to the CDC, persistent pressure or pain in the chest is a symptom of COVID-19 and 210 survey participants claim to continue feeling this symptom after the virus is gone. As a respiratory virus, it's possible that this pain or pressure is actually being felt in the lungs. However, according to *Diagnostic and Interventional Cardiology*, stroke, heart failure, arrhythmias, and other cardiac events have also been linked to coronavirus so sufferers should take this **lingering symptom seriously.**

50- **Decrease in taste** A loss of sense of taste is a common symptom of COVID-19 but 221 survey respondents claim the virus may have completely changed their sense of taste. According to Kaiser Permanente, a loss of sense of taste or partial loss may cause tastes to change. These changes may also be caused by a decrease in taste buds or changes in the way the nervous system processes certain taste sensations

51- **Tinnitus** is a ringing or noise in the ear and 233 survey respondents claim they now experience this ringing or humming in the ears after recovering from COVID-19. According to the American Tinnitus Association, the onset of tinnitus may occur due to stress and anxiety, after there's been damage to the inner ear, or when other conditions or diseases are developed.

52- **Neurological damage** According to a study published in the Elsevier Public Health Emergency Collection, "Viral infections have detrimental impacts on neurological functions, and even cause severe neurological damage." 243 survey participants reported feeling nerve sensations after COVID-19, which may be due to neurological damage caused by the virus.

53- **Constant thirst** When you contract an illness or a virus like coronavirus, your body's working overtime to fight it. According to the Mayo Clinic, your body needs more fluids when you're sick and if it doesn't get the fluids, you're likely to suffer from constant thirst. It's your body's way of telling you it's not getting enough fluids to continue fighting and recovering from the virus

54- **Mucous membranes** in some COVID-19 cases, patients have developed rashes on their skin. According to a research letter published in the *JAMA Network*, some coronavirus patients suffered from enanthem, a skin rash that looks like small white spots on the mucous membranes. Other patients had widespread urticaria, or hives, on their skin. Other rashes were also found in some COVID-19 patients who were studied. Scientists aren't sure if this side effect is directly related to the virus or attributed to certain medications

55- **Flashes of light** According to UCLA Health, "floaters" are little specks or lines that float around in your field of vision occasionally. If you constantly see floaters or they're accompanied by flashes of light, it may indicate you have a retina tear or vitreous detachment, which occurs when vitreous gel in the eye separates from the retina. In the survey, 249 respondents claimed to suffer from floaters or flashes of light in their vision after COVID-19.

56- **Back pain** as with most illnesses, coronavirus is associated with muscle aches and pains. Patients with COVID-19 who were bedridden or spent an extended period inactive may experience upper back pain due to immobility. According to Kaiser Permanente, upper back pain isn't as common as lower back pain but may be caused by muscle strain, poor posture, or pressure on the spinal nerves

57- **Fatigue** is a common symptom of coronavirus, but some sufferers are having trouble shaking off that tiredness. According to an article published in *The Scientist*, it's possible that COVID-19 may lead to chronic illness, including chronic fatigue. Scientists are tracking these symptoms amongst sufferers who seek treatment so they can get a grasp on what other symptoms may lead to chronic illness.

58- **Anxiety** According to Northwestern Medicine, tremors may be caused by stress, anxiety, or too much caffeine. Tremors or shakes when you pick up a glass of water or hold a piece of paper may also indicate that you have essential tremor (ET), which is a neurological disorder that causes these shakes. These tremors may occur because the body is recovering from the stress of the virus, they may indicate ET, or there may be another underlying cause.

59- **Dehydrating** According to the University of Rochester Medical Center, muscle cramps usually occur after heavy exercise, when you're experiencing muscle fatigue, or if your body's dehydrated. Since the virus and other illnesses are notorious for dehydrating your body and causing muscle fatigue, these calf cramps may be an explainable symptom of coronavirus. Massaging, stretching, and warm compresses could help mitigate these cramps.

60- **Itchy, dry, and red eyes** An article published in *Review of Optometry* reviewed the relationship between ocular symptoms and coronavirus in Chinese patients. It found that 27% of those studied complained of itchy, dry, and red eyes. Some even began to develop sore and dry eyes a few days before any other COVID-19 symptoms. Researchers feel this may be because coronavirus "infects the mucosa membrane epithelium and even lymphocytes, which are both abundant in ocular surface tissue."

61- **Ear pain, muffled hearing, or dizziness** According to the Mayo Clinic, when your ears are clogged "your eustachian tubes — which run between your middle ear and the back of your nose — become obstructed." It may cause pressure, ear pain, muffled hearing, or dizziness. The survey found that 267 participants experienced clogged ears as a long-lasting symptom of COVID-19. Since clogged ears are common with a stuffy nose and other respiratory illnesses or sinus infections, it's a common symptom of coronavirus. To relieve pressure, you can try popping your ears or taking a nasal decongestant.

62- **Nausea or vomiting** While it's not usually listed as a common symptom of COVID-19, many who got the virus also suffered from nausea, vomiting, diarrhea, or other gastrointestinal problems. The survey found that 314 respondents claimed they still suffered from nausea or vomiting after coronavirus. According to the Mayo Clinic, these gastrointestinal symptoms were varied and some felt them well before a diagnosis. Others only dealt with these symptoms for one day.

63- **Shortness of breath** is a common symptom of COVID-19, but 318 survey participants reported that they continued to feel shortness of breath or exhaustion when they bent over. According to Penn Medicine, this may be a sign of an ongoing pulmonary problem or heart problem. While shortness of breath is common with COVID-19 sufferers, those who have recovered should seek medical attention if this symptom doesn't seem to be going away.

64- **Myalgia** COVID-19 causes myalgia, pain in a muscle or a group of muscles. An article published in *Nature Public Health Emergency Collection* concludes that myalgia in COVID-19 patients lingers longer than it may with other illnesses. Lower back pain is usually associated with pneumonia or poor lung function and since COVID-19 is a respiratory virus, it makes sense that patients are more likely to experience this type of muscle pain.

65- **Gastrointestinal** While not a common symptom of COVID-19, many who contracted the virus did report gastrointestinal problems. This could explain why 344 survey respondents reported dealing with abdominal pain well after contracting the virus. In a study published through the American Gastrological Association, 31.9% of COVID-19 patients studied claimed to have gastrointestinal problems associated with the virus.

66- **While a dry cough** is most associated with coronavirus, some patients may experience phlegm in the back of their throat during the later stages. For coronavirus patients dealing with phlegm, the University of Maryland Medical System suggests taking an expectorant to help get the mucus out and make your cough more productive. Staying hydrated and drinking warm beverages may also help to break up the phlegm

67- **Loss of taste, called ageusia**, and loss of smell, called anosmia, are common symptoms of the virus and the duration of these symptoms varies by patient. A study published in the *Journal of Korean Medical Science* analyzed Korean COVID-19 sufferers and the duration of this specific symptom. The study found that, "Most patients with anosmia or ageusia recovered within 3 weeks."

**68- Heartburn** occurs when stomach acid backs up into the tube that carries food from your mouth to your stomach (esophagus)," according to the Mayo Clinic. Since the virus is known to cause gastrointestinal problems, some patients may take longer to recover from these inconsistencies than others. Avoiding alcohol, spicy foods, and large meals may help curb these long-lasting symptoms.

**69- Neuropathy is weakness or numbness due to nerve damage. Since the virus can do some** damage to the nervous system, this may be a lingering symptom for some sufferers. According to a report published in the Elsevier Public Health Emergency Collection, COVID-19 may even disguise itself as motor peripheral neuropathy without other symptoms. Nerve fibers may be more sensitive when a patient is infected with the virus, causing this numbing of the hands and feet.

**70- Sadness** As a pandemic, COVID-19 sufferers are required to quarantine, which may mean isolating from loved ones and not being able to engage in activities they enjoy. A study published in The Lancet analyzed mental side effects of the virus and concluded that medical professionals should watch their patients for signs of depression or some neuropsychiatric syndromes well after recovery.

**71- Congested or Runny Nose** According to the American Pharmacists Association, the CDC recently added "runny nose" as a symptom of COVID-19. 414 survey respondents claimed a congested or runny nose as a lingering symptom of the virus. A runny nose is one way to get rid of the mucus in your body after the virus, so it may persist until the mucus is gone.

**72- Blurry Vision** Blurry vision may be a sign of nerve damage or may also occur when other COVID-19 symptoms are going strong, such as a fever or headache. According to the American Academy of Ophthalmology, blurred vision may also be a symptom of endophthalmitis, which is an infection of tissue or fluids inside the eye. If this is the case, quick treatment is required to prevent blindness.

**73- Hair Loss** According to Dr. Shilpi Harpal, MD from the Cleveland Clinic, hair loss isn't necessarily a symptom of COVID-19 but may be a side effect of the virus. She states, "We are seeing patients who had COVID-19 two to three months ago and are now experiencing hair loss." In the survey, 423 respondents reported experiencing hair loss after coronavirus. Dr. Khetarpal says this may be due to a change in diet, high fever, extreme weight loss, or any other "shock to the system" that COVID-19 may have caused.

74- **Chills** The CDC conducted a study on coronavirus patients and found that 96% of patients recovered from chills and 97% recovered from fever. While most recovered from all COVID-19 symptoms, 34% still revealed that they were suffering from one or more lasting symptoms when interviewed four to eight days after testing positive. 65% of sufferers returned to their usual state of health around seven days after testing positive but chronic medical conditions, age, weight, gender, and other factors may affect how long symptoms, such as fever and chills, last.

75- **Tachycardia** According to the Mayo Clinic, tachycardia occurs when your heart beats over 100 beats per minute. It's a form of arrhythmia, or a heartbeat disorder. In the survey, 448 respondents experienced tachycardia after suffering from COVID-19. It may be the body's response to stress, trauma, or illness. However, if tachycardia is left untreated and continues to occur, it can lead to serious complications, such as heart failure or stroke.

76- **Partial or Complete Loss of Sense of Smell** Partial or complete loss of sense of smell is a common symptom with COVID-19 and many other respiratory viruses, according to Penn Medicine. Since your olfactory system is so close to your respiratory system, virus cells can enter nerve and receptor cells and cause damage. It can take a long time for these cells to repair and some cells may never fully recover from the virus.

77- **Night Sweats** According to Kaiser Permanente, night sweats are different from regular sweating because they occur only at night and include intense sweating, enough to soak through your clothes and sheets. It's possible that night sweats are present due to a residual fever, but they may also be caused by thyroid level issues, menopause, anxiety, or infections. New medication or other lingering symptoms, such as chills and muscle aches, may also contribute to long- lasting night sweats.

78- **Sore Throat** While not all coronavirus sufferers experience a sore throat, it's one of the common symptoms the CDC lists for the virus. According to the CDC, viruses and infections cause sore throats, which may be why this is a lingering symptom for some coronavirus patients.

79- **Diarrhea** While it's not the most common, diarrhea is listed by the CDC as a symptom of COVID-19. A study conducted by several researchers analyzed 206 patients with low severity COVID-19 and 48 experienced digestive problems first before other coronavirus symptoms. Diarrhea lasted an average of 14 days for COVID-19 patients in the study.

80- **Heart Palpitations** Even after the fever, headache, and dry cough have disappeared, some patients who have "recovered" from COVID-19 may experience heart palpitations. A study published in *JAMA Cardiology* examined 100 recovered COVID-19 patients and found that 78 of them had "cardiac involvement" while 60% had ongoing myocardial inflammation. Ongoing heart issues, such as palpitations, may be long-lasting for COVID-19 patients, regardless of their illness severity.

81- **Joint Pain** Dr. Richard Deem from Cedars- Sinai explains that as your immune system attempts to fight off COVID-19 or any type of illness, white blood cells produce interleukins to help join the fight. While these interleukins are useful in fighting off the virus cells, they also cause muscle and joint pain. The immune response may still be heightened in these recovering patients, causing this joint pain to last.

82- **Cough** A lingering cough can be a side effect of any type of cold, flu, or illness. According to a study conducted by the World Health Organization (WHO) on Chinese COVID-19 patients, 61.7% developed a dry cough. As a respiratory virus, the cough associated with COVID-19 may take a long time to go away because your body is attempting to get rid of lingering mucus and phlegm.

83- **Persistent Chest Pain or Pressure** Chest pain or pressure was a common lingering COVID-19 symptom among survey participants. Since coronavirus affects the lungs and respiratory system, this chest pain may be attributed to the virus still settling in the body. According to the Mayo Clinic, sudden, sharp chest pains are referred to as pleurisy and it may indicate that the lung walls are inflamed. Pleurisy may be a sign of pneumonia or another type of infection, so recovered COVID-19 patients should see a doctor if this symptom persists.

84- **Dizziness** COVID-19 is a respiratory virus that also has nervous system side effects. According to a study published in the *Journal of the American College of Emergency Physicians Open*, "symptoms including headache, dizziness, vertigo, and paresthesia have been reported." This may be due to decreased oxygen levels, dehydration, fevers, or headaches also caused by the virus.

85- **Memory Problems** A paper published in the *Journal of Alzheimer's Disease* analyzes potential long-term neurological effects of COVID-19 on patients who experienced severe cases. Memory problems and cognitive decline are potential side effects for some of these patients. Since the virus affects the nervous system, memory problems may be a lingering side effect for some patients, especially those who suffered severe cases.

86- **Anxiety** According to a poll conducted by the American Psychiatric Association, about 36% of Americans feel coronavirus has had a serious impact on their mental health. Between quarantining, social isolation, and worry about developing a severe case of coronavirus, it's no wonder anxiety is a lingering symptom for COVID-19 patients.

87- **Difficulty Sleeping** Sleep is crucial because it keeps the immune system functioning properly, heightens brain function, stabilizes mood, and improves mental health. 782 survey respondents claimed they were having difficulty sleeping, even after recovering from COVID-19. This lack of sleep may be due to anxiety or worry about the virus or may be attributed to other lingering symptoms, such as muscle pain or cough. Setting specific bedtimes and only using your bed for sleep may help with these difficulties.

88- **Headache** According to Dr. Sandhya Mela with the Hartford HealthCare Headache Center,

"It is estimated that headache is a symptom of COVID-19 in about 13% of patients with COVID-19. It is the fifth most common COVID-19 symptom after fever, cough, muscle aches, and trouble breathing." In the survey, 902 participants claimed that a headache was a long- lasting symptom after COVID-19. This may be due to dehydration, congestion, or other symptoms of coronavirus, such as a fever.

89- **Inability to Exercise or Be Active** After recovering from COVID-19, some patients find it hard to exercise or be active, even if they were fit before contracting the virus. 916 survey participants reported that they were still unable to exercise after recovering from coronavirus. According to a study published in *JAMA Cardiology*, researchers recommend that patients who suffered from severe cases of COVID-19 wait at least two weeks before resuming light exercise. This allows time for doctors to see if heart or lung conditions develop that could make it dangerous to engage in physical activity.

90- **Difficulty Concentrating or Focusing** The long-term effects of COVID-19 are unknown since the virus is so new, but researchers are seeing certain neurological effects on patients who have recovered. Studies conducted in Wuhan analyzed these neurological conditions and found that 40% of the patients analyzed experienced confusion and conscious disturbance. This is commonly referred to as "brain fog" and many patients express feeling this way while recovering from coronavirus.

91- **Muscle or Body Aches** Body aches are a common symptom of many illnesses, including coronavirus. In this survey, 1,048 participants reported feeling these body aches after their COVID-19 diagnosis. According to Dr. Tania Elliott, MD FAAAAI, FACAAI, "Your body aches when you have the flu because your immune system is revving up to fight infection." It's not necessarily the virus that causes these aches but your body's own reaction to the virus invasion.

92- **Fatigue** Fatigue was the most common lingering symptom of coronavirus. WHO study

# Section Eight Long Hauler Symptoms Diagnosis

**8.0 OMICRON and DELTA** viruses can invade and infect multi-system

H. Brain and Neurological System COVID Related Symptoms
I. Cardiovascular system COVID Related Symptoms
J. Respiratory System COVID Related Symptoms
K. Liver COVID Related Symptoms
L. Renal COVID Related Symptoms
M. Gastrointestinal system COVID Related Symptoms
N. Endocrine Systems COVID Related Symptoms

## 8.1 Neurological Disorder Long Symptoms

Since the virus can gain entry to the brain via olfactory and make its way to the brain, in this section we will discuss neurological disorder as many posts COVID-19 and delta virus's infection patients are reporting one or many symptoms as listed in the table below:

**Table nine**: Neurological Disorder Long Hauler Symptoms

| Symptoms of fatigue include: |
| --- |
| doing tasks in the wrong order |
| finding it increasingly difficult to perform more than one task at once |
| forgetting to do things often |
| working on automatic and not thinking |
| falling asleep for small amounts of time |
| feeling tired or yawning all the time |
| being more irritable than usual |
| being frustrated by tasks |
| having difficulty concentrating |
| being uncommunicative |
| Headaches |
| Sleep disturbances |
| Anxiety, depression, and stress post-COVID |

### 8.1.1  Recommended Diagnosis & imaging to isolate the problem

Note: All imaging in this document is for illustration only and physician recommendations is advised

1- Cerebrospinal fluid (CSF) leaks diagnose
2- Inflammation in and around your brain
3- Brain Infarct area
4- Brain Inflammation and Arteries Blockage
5- Brain Scan Blood Clots
6- Brain Flairs and any lesions, nodular growth

### 8.1.2  Imaging for cerebrospinal fluid leakage

Your doctor will perform a history and <u>physical exam</u>. Often, the doctor will examine your nose with an endoscope. Your doctor may also ask you to lean forward for several minutes to see if drainage comes out your nose. If the drainage can be collected, it is often sent for laboratory testing to confirm that it is cerebrospinal fluid.

**Figure six:** MRI Scan for Cerebrospinal Fluid

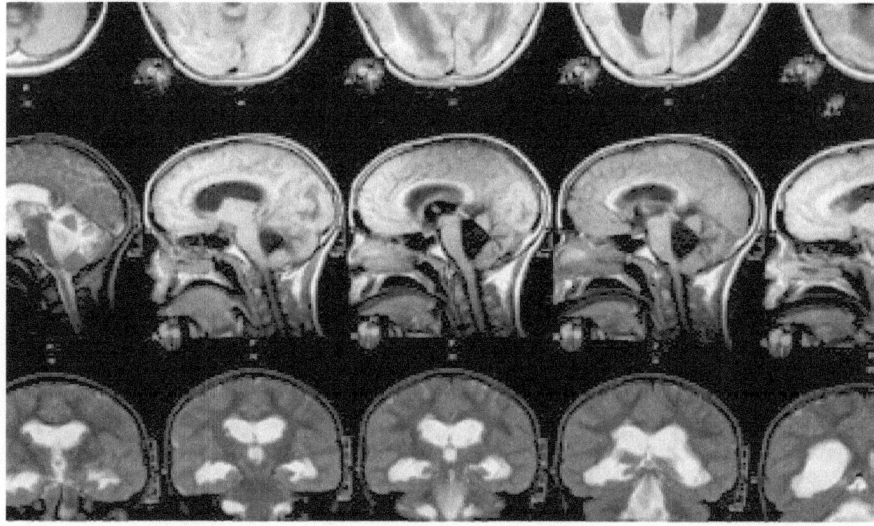

**Figure seven:** Cerebrospinal Fluid Illustration Anatomy

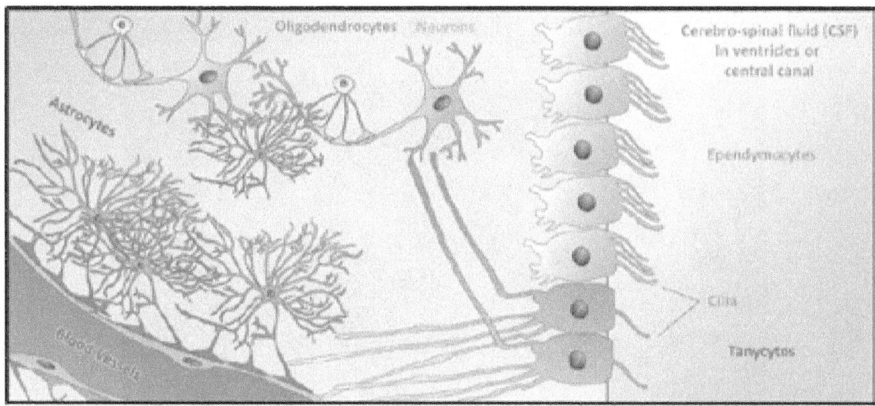

### 8.1.3 Evidence of Inflammation That Causes Neurological Disorder

**Figure eight:** MRI scan, Brain Inflammation as Results from COVID Infection

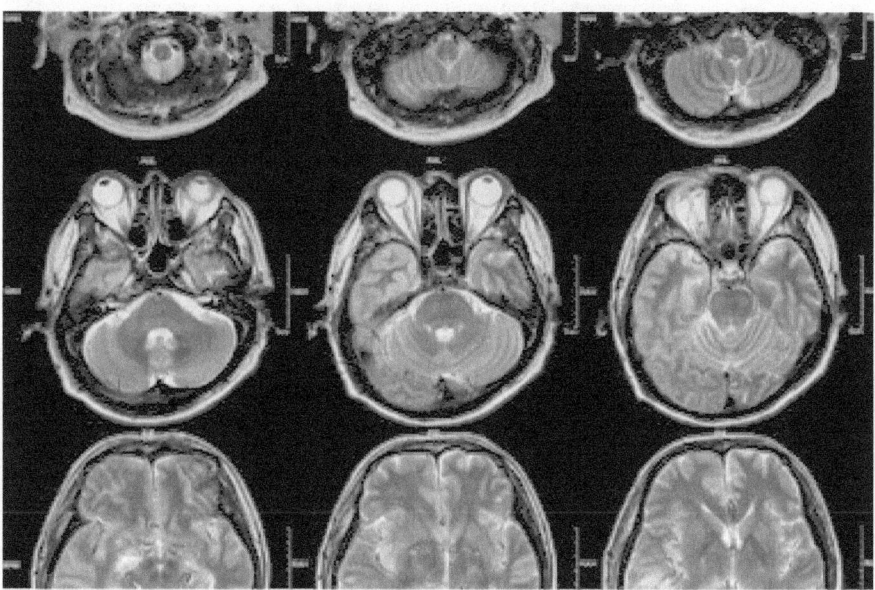

## 8.1.4 Evidence of any Infarct Area

**Figure nine:** CT Scan Brain Infarct area

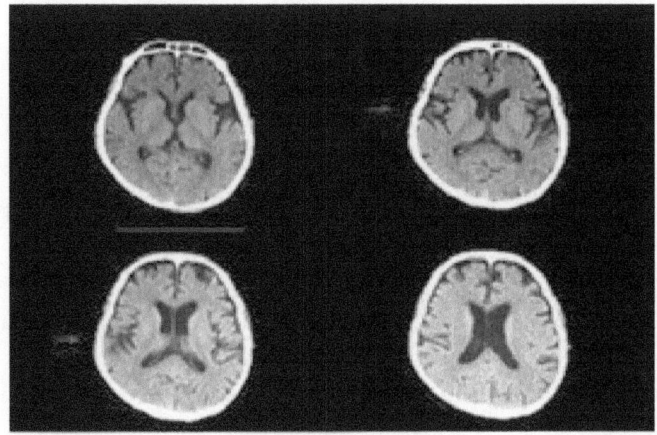

**Figure ten:** CT Scan Brain Infarct area

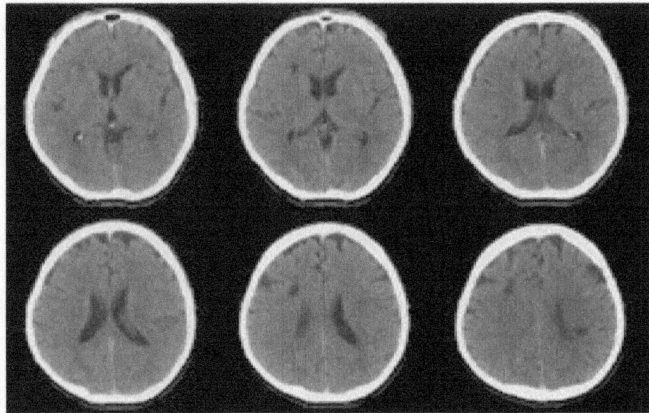

## 8.1.5   Evidence of any blockage

**Figure eleven:** MRI Scan Brain Inflammation and Arteries Blockage

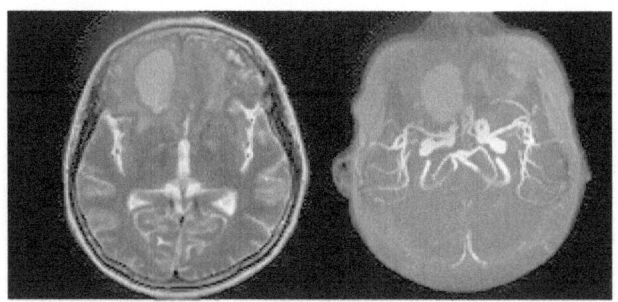

**Figure twelve: MRI** Multi Brain slides defining damages and infarct in different areas of the brain

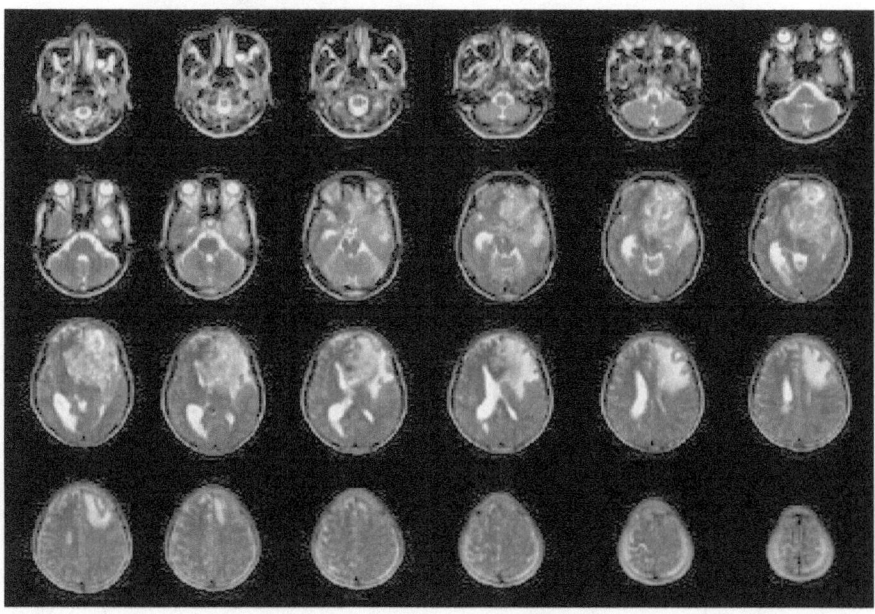

### 8.1.6 Blood Blockage Areas

**Figure thirteen:** Brain Scan Slide Two Demonstrate symmetric diffuse T2/FLAIR hyperintensity

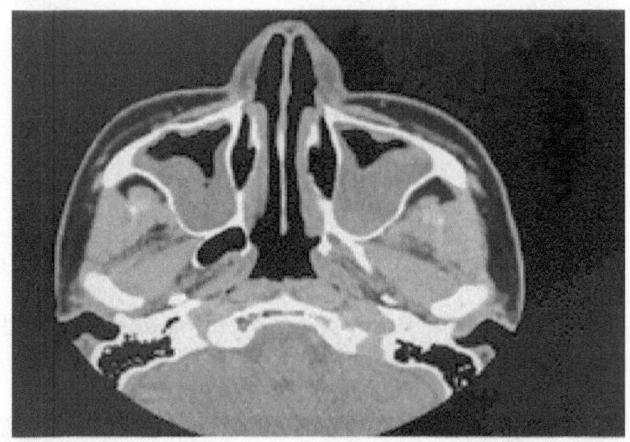

**Figure fourteen:** Brain Flairs and any lesions, nodular growth

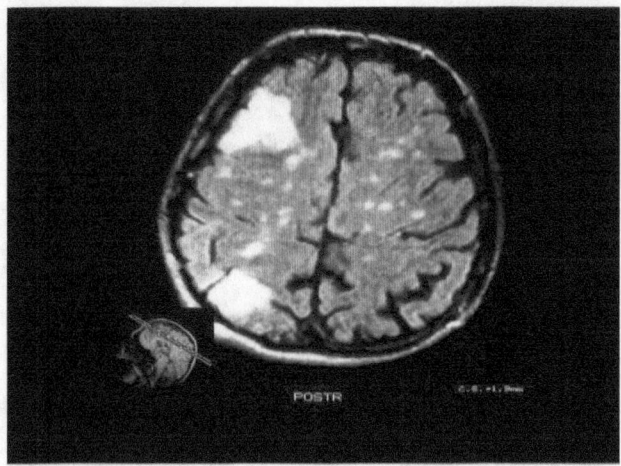

### 8.1.7 Brain Scan Blood Clots as Results COVID Infection and Immune system Storm

**Figure fifteen:** Blood clots and brain damaged area can be caused by Immune Cytokine Storm in response of COVID infection

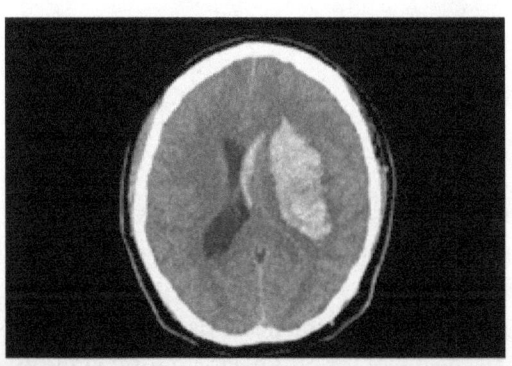

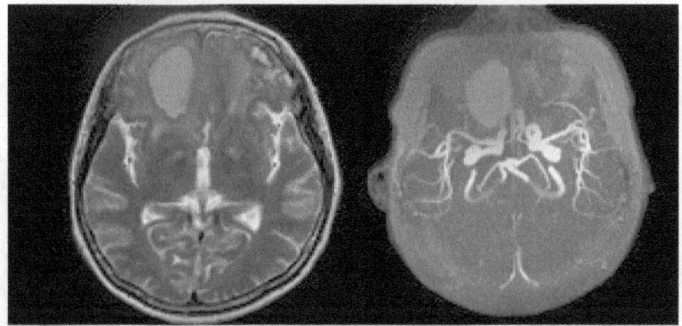

## 8.2 Cardiovascular System COVID Related Symptoms

In this section we will discuss Cardiovascular system disorder as many posts COVID-19 and delta virus's infection patients are reporting one or more symptoms as listed in the table below:

**Table ten:** Cardiovascular System Symptoms

| Cardiovascular System Symptoms Results from Previous COVID Infection |
| --- |
| Heartbeat Rapidly |
| Palpitation |
| Lightheaded |
| Chest Discomfort |
| Postural Tachycardia |

**8.2.1 SARS-CoV-2**, the virus that causes COVID-19, most commonly affects the lungs but It can also lead to serious heart problems. Lung damage caused by the virus prevents oxygen from reaching the heart muscle, which in turn damages the heart tissue and prevents it from getting oxygen to other tissues. Doctor will perform vital signs exam and perform ECG to determine your heart health including MRI.

**Figure sixteen:** MRI showing heart left ventricle infarct Area

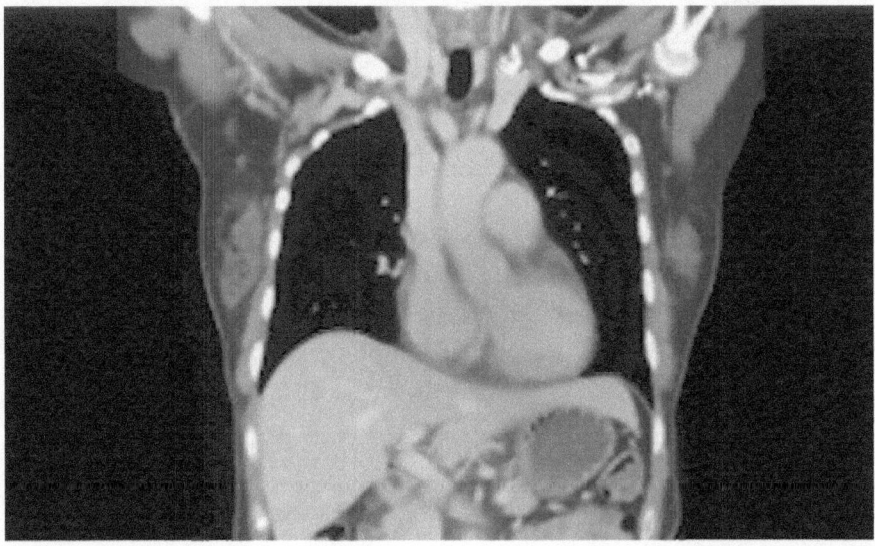

**Figure seventeen**: ECG diagnosis ST segment elevation and depression

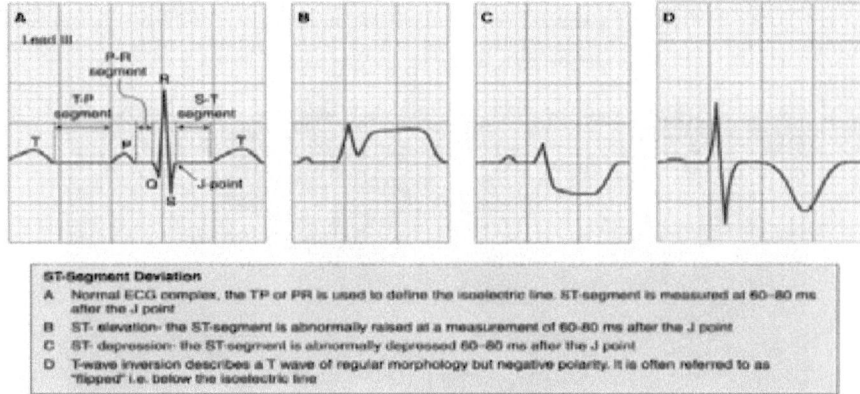

ST-Segment Deviation
A  Normal ECG complex, the TP or PR is used to define the isoelectric line. ST-segment is measured at 60–80 ms after the J point
B  ST- elevation- the ST-segment is abnormally raised at a measurement of 60-80 ms after the J point
C  ST- depression- the ST-segment is abnormally depressed 60–80 ms after the J point
D  T-wave inversion describes a T wave of regular morphology but negative polarity. It is often referred to as "flipped" i.e. below the isoelectric line

## 8.3    Respiratory System COVID Related Symptoms

In this section we will discuss pulmonary system disorder as many posts OMICRON and delta virus's infection patients are reporting one or more symptoms as listed in the table below:

**Table eleven:** Respiratory Symptoms

| Respiratory | |
|---|---|
| 1- | longer-term symptoms include: |
| 2- | Fatigue |
| 3- | Shortness of breath |
| 4- | Cough |
| 5- | Joint pain |
| 6- | Chest pain |
| 7- | Muscle pain |
| 8- | Headaches |
| 9- | Fast or pounding heartbeat |
| 10 | Intermittent fever |

**8.3.1   Doctor will perform vital signs exam** including Oxygen level followed by MRI imaging to determine the severity of lungs damage as results of post COVID infection due to low oxygen level during the infection and virus infection damages of the alveolar.

**Figure eighteen**: Lung's infection and fluid detected

Chest Xray film of a patient with pneumonia at left lower lung. SARS-CoV-2 virus covid-19 infection.

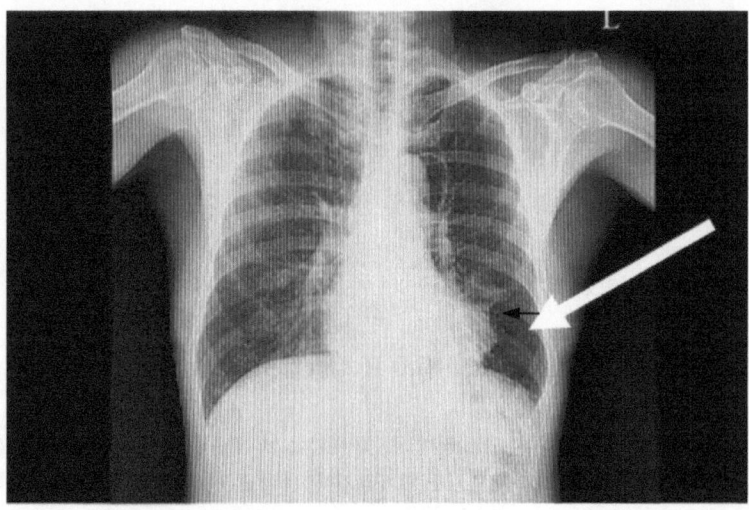

A chest Xray film of a patient with right middle and lower lobes pneumonia, left lower lobe pneumonia, and left middle lung nodule. SARS-CoV-2 virus covid-19 infection.

**Figure nineteen**: lower lobes pneumonia

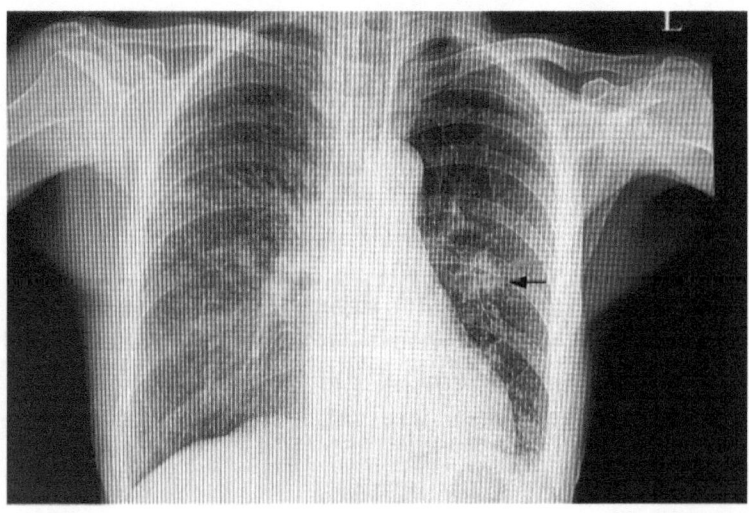

**Figure twenty:** Sever lungs damage for COVID 19 deceased persons

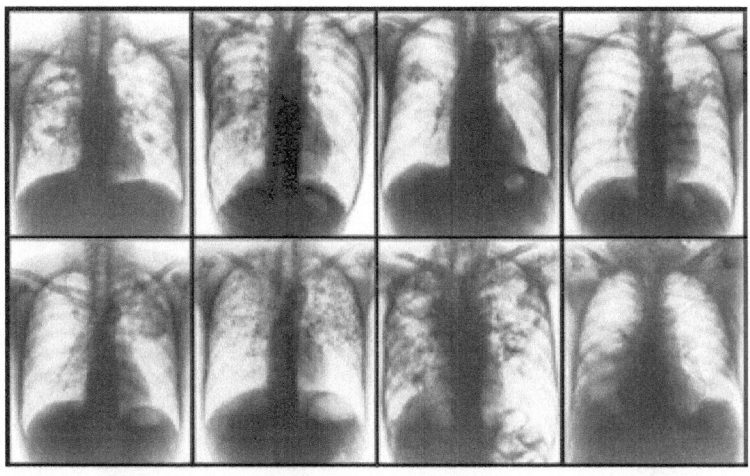

**Figure twenty-one:** Lungs upper right mid lobe damage

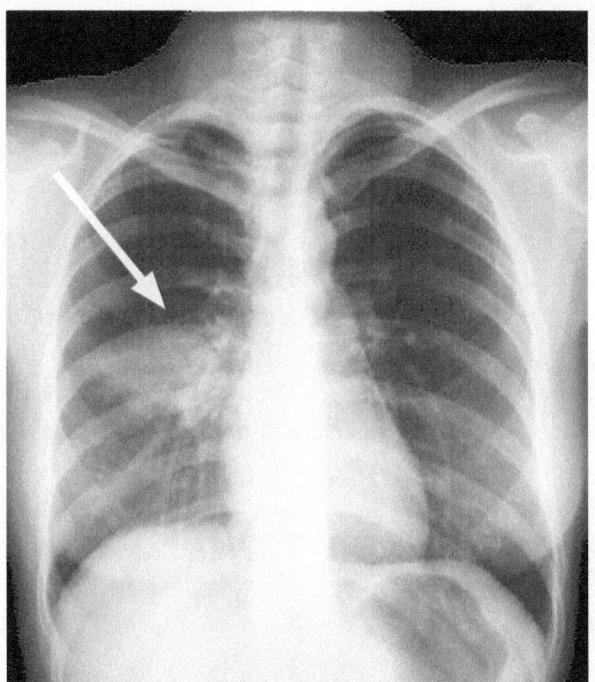

### 8.4 kidney impairment as results of COVID 19 infection

In this section we will discuss renal system kidney disorder as many posts COVID-19 and delta virus's infection patients are reporting one or more symptoms as listed in the table below:

**Table twelve:** Renal System Symptoms

| Kidney Symptoms |
| --- |
| Not peeing enough. |
| Swelling in ankles, legs, and around eyes. |
| Tiredness. |
| Shortness of breath. |
| Feeling confused. |
| Nausea. |
| Seizures or coma. |
| Chest pressure or pain. |

Recently reported that some COVID-19 patients had an elevated level of proteinuria, suggesting **SARS-CoV-2 infection** might result in acute kidney injury (AKI)[17]. SARS-CoV-2 can also directly infect human kidney organoids via the ACE2 receptor[18] **Doctor will perform vital signs exam** including Oxygen level followed by MRI imaging to determine the severity of kidney damage in case of low oxygen level detection and sever COVID infection

### 8.4.1    Renal Diagnosis

*UACR urine test*

An early way to find out if you may have chronic kidney disease (CKD) is by taking a UACR (urine albumin-to-creatinine ratio) test once a year. A UACR test can detect how much small protein, called **albumin**, is in the urine, which is one of the earliest indicators of CKD or kidney damage. A damaged kidney can't filter as well as it should and lets some protein pass into the urine. A healthy kidney doesn't let any protein pass into the urine.

A UACR urine test isn't always part of a routine health screening and is different from usual urinalysis tests that are commonly used at doctor appointments, so be sure to ask your healthcare provider specifically for a UACR urine test.

**Figure twenty-two:** Kidney impairments

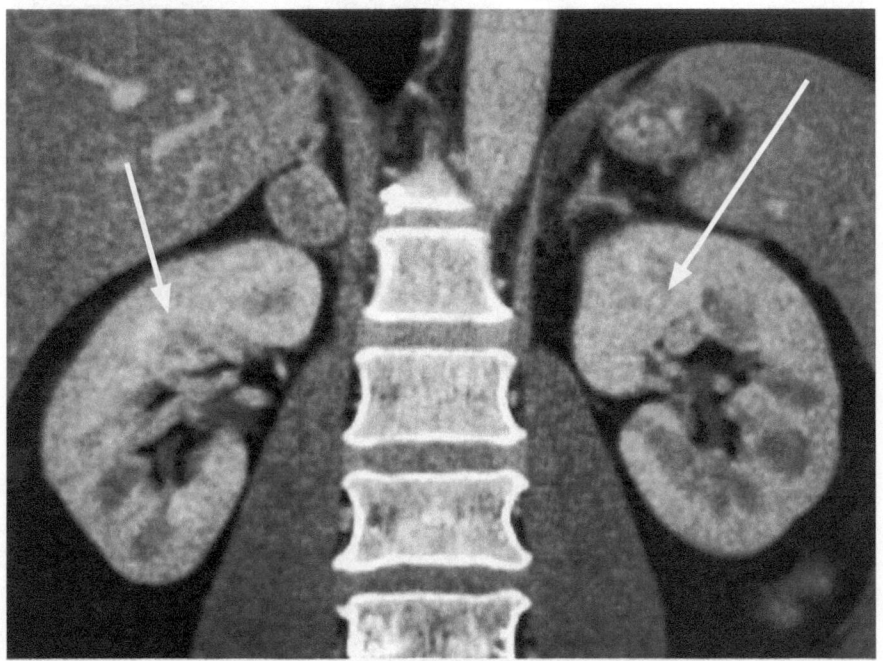

**Figure twenty-three:** Kidney Infarct CT and MRI Imaging

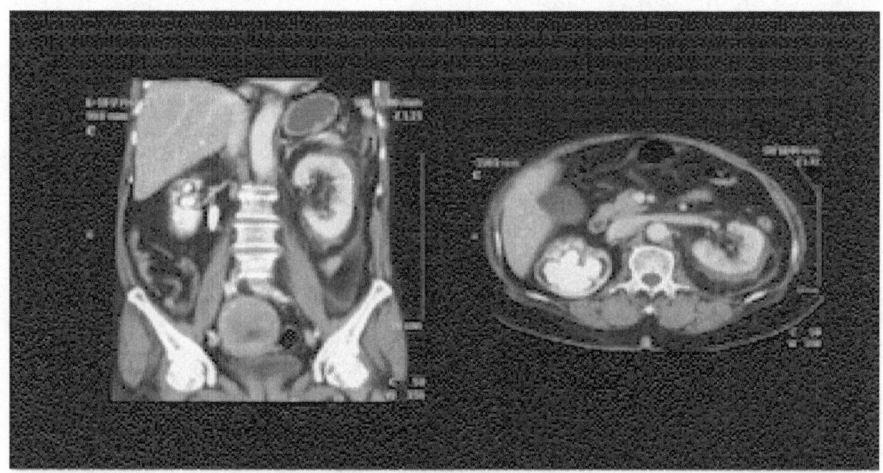

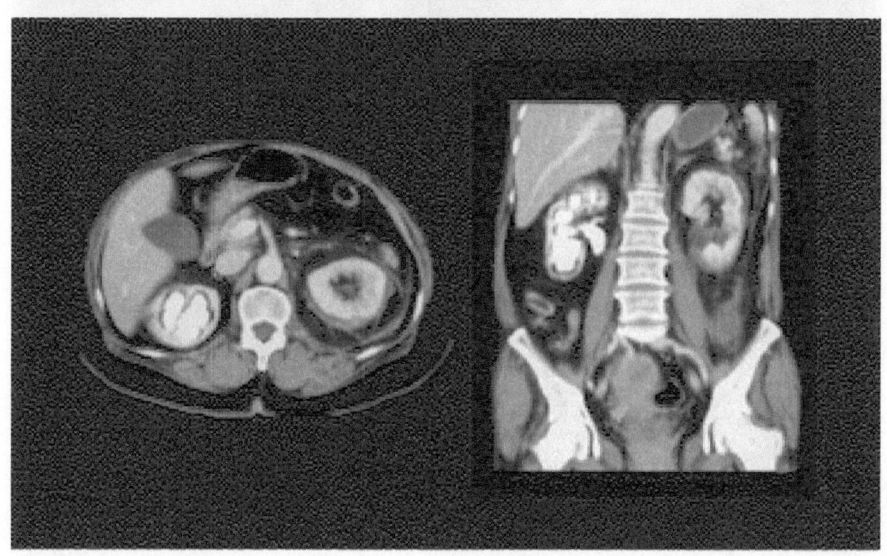

## 8.5 Endocrine System

The pathogenesis of COVID-19 entails entry of SARS-CoV-2 via the respiratory system and lodgment in the lung parenchyma. Thereafter, it uses angiotensin-converting enzyme 2 (ACE2) as a receptor for ingress into host cell.

ACE2 expressed in other tissues. As a matter of fact, several endocrine organs do express ACE2, namely pancreas, thyroid, testis, ovary, adrenal glands, and pituitary. Even though one could expect endocrine repercussions due to interaction of SARS-CoV-2 with ACE2 expressed on these organs, COVID-19 and Endocrine Pancreas

ACE2 is expressed in pancreas with mRNA levels being higher in pancreas than in the lungs. The expression is seen on the exocrine pancreas as well as on the islets. Exocrine pancreatic injury is manifested

COVID-19 could also lead to worsening of insulin resistance in patients with pre-existing type 2 diabetes mellitus (T2DM). Apart from inducing a plethora of cytokines, SARS-CoV2 increases serum levels of fetuin A, glycoprotein.

### 8.5.1   COVID-19 and the hypothalamus–pituitary

Neurological manifestations do occur in patients with COVID-19 and include, among others, hyposmia. Expression of ACE2 by the olfactory epithelial supporting cells could explain much of these olfactory symptoms. The portal of entry of the virus into the central nervous system (CNS) and pituitary tissues do express ACE2 and can theoretically be the viral targets. In fact,

### 8.5.2   COVID-19 and thyroid

Data on thyroid involvement by coronavirus is most scarce. A study had reported that serum T3 and T4 levels were lower in patients with SARS as compared to controls both during the acute and convalescent phases. This could simply imply an underlying thyroid syndrome

**Figure Twenty-four: Endocrine System Diagram**

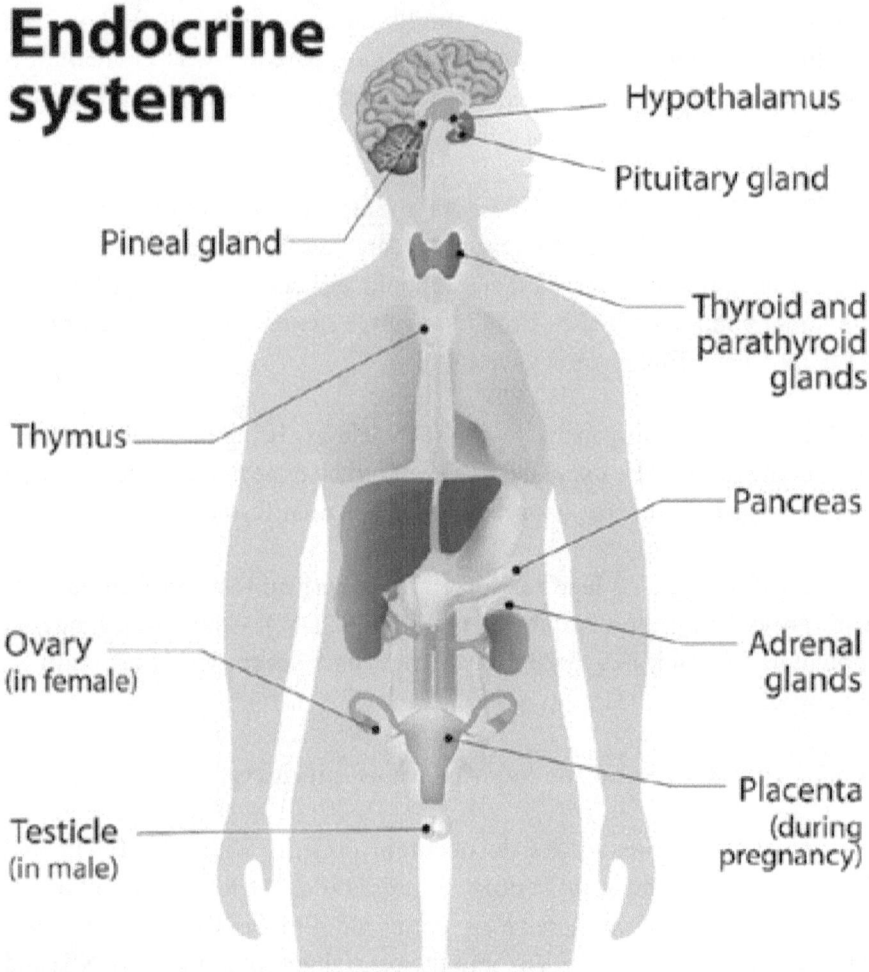

### 8.5.3 Acute Liver Injury in Covid Patient

Expressed in tissues during the viral replication cycle and causes inflammation in most tissues, including the liver. This inflammatory response facilitates viral clearance from the tissues and promotes an adaptive immune response to viral infection. CD4+ lymphocytes promote the transformation of B cells into plasma cells and enhance antibody production. Cytotoxic T lymphocytes are active in most tissues, which reflects an effective antiviral response, but may also cause extensive liver tissue injury.

### 8.5.4 The thyroid and COVID-19

COVID 19 infections can causes decrease in the FT3, FT4, and TSH levels. Further discovery is underway

### 8.5.5 Adrenal insufficiency

COVID-19 pandemic may be a new reason for patient and physician concern. Adrenal insufficiency may confer a potentially increased risk of acquiring COVID-19 infection, as this condition is associated to an impaired natural immunity function, with a defective action of neutrophils and natural killer-cells.

### 8.6 Liver Damage of post COVID 19 infections

**Table thirteen: Liver Symptoms**

| Liver Symptoms |
|---|
| Skin and eyes that appear yellowish (jaundice) |
| Abdominal pain and swelling. |
| Swelling in the legs and ankles. |
| Itchy skin. |
| Dark urine color. |
| Pale stool color. |
| Chronic fatigue. |
| Nausea or vomiting. |

**8.6.1** The spectrum of liver injury in COVID-19 may range from direct infection by SARS-CoV-2 entering the AC2 receptors or indirect involvement by systemic inflammation, hypoxic changes, iatrogenic causes such as drugs and ventilation to exacerbation of underlying liver disease

**Figure Twenty-five:** Liver Inflammation MRI Scan

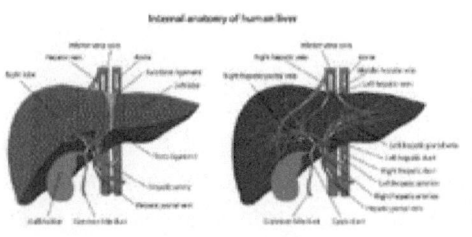 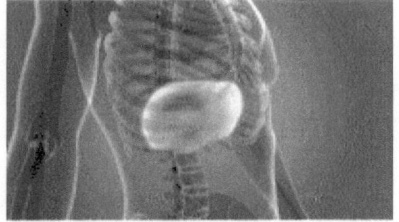

**8.6.2** **One possible mechanism** for the liver injury observed in patients with COVID-19 is direct hepatic infection by SARS-CoV-2. The SARS-CoV-2 host cell receptor is angiotensin-converting enzyme 2 (ACE2),(18) and SARS-CoV-2 cellular entry also involves transmembrane serine protease 2 (TMPRSS2)

**Figure Twenty-six**: CT Scan Liver tissues damage as results previous COVID Infection

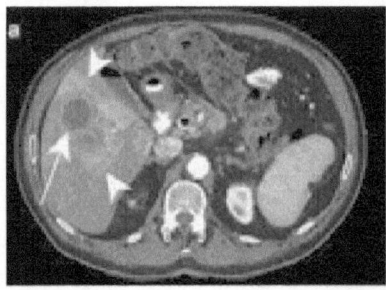 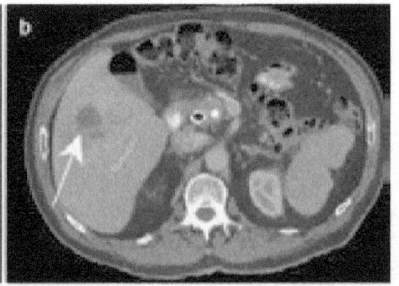

Pyogenic abscess in an old male patient with a history of chronic pancreatitis who presented with asthenia and fever. Axial arterial phase (a) and portal venous phase (b) contrast-enhanced CT show small clustering lesions with a dominant hypoattenuating lesion in segment V of the liver (white arrows) corresponding to pyogenic hepatic abscesses. Altered perfusion disorder is observed as geographic areas of hyper attenuation peripheral to the h1epatic abscesses

## 8.7 Gastrointestinal System Diagnosis

Studies have found evidence that the coronavirus can infect the digestive system, including the pancreas, which regulates blood sugar. The evidence includes finding viral RNA in human feces, imaging scans showing bowel abnormalities, a correlation between digestive symptoms and a positive stool test,

**Table fourteen: Gastrointestinal** Symptoms

| GI Symptoms |
| --- |
| lack of appetite |
| lack of smell or taste |
| diarrhea |
| nausea |
| vomiting up blooding |
| nausea, vomiting, or both |
| abdominal pain |
| acid reflux |
| colitis |
| Reduce intestinal movement |

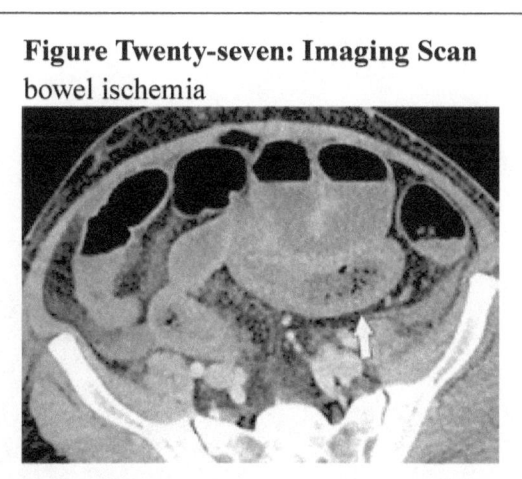

**Figure Twenty-seven: Imaging Scan** bowel ischemia

## 8.7.1 Gastrointestinal System

Symptoms he most prevalent symptom is the loss of appetite or anorexia. Which is second most common is upper-abdominal or epigastric (the area right below your ribs) pain or diarrhea, and that has happened with about 20 percent of patients with COVID-19. As indication COVID 19 made its way to infect upper abdominal system.

As noticed mucosal cells of **the lower intestine can be infected by other coronaviruses**, resulting in diarrhea and other enteric symptoms. In this case, SARS-CoV-2 could be carried by saliva and secretions into the digestive tract, where it would infect the ACE2-expressing enterocytes.

**Figure twenty-eight:** COVID infection of small bowel

# Mesenteric ischemia

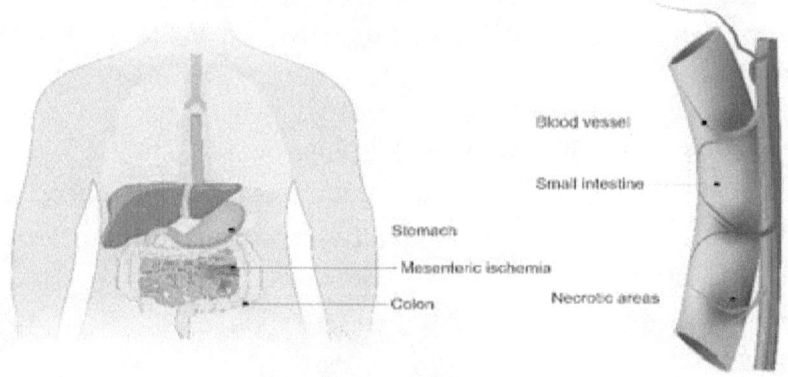

# MULTI ORGAN SYMPTOMS COVID 19 RELATED CHART

## *Summary of Long Hauler Symptoms*

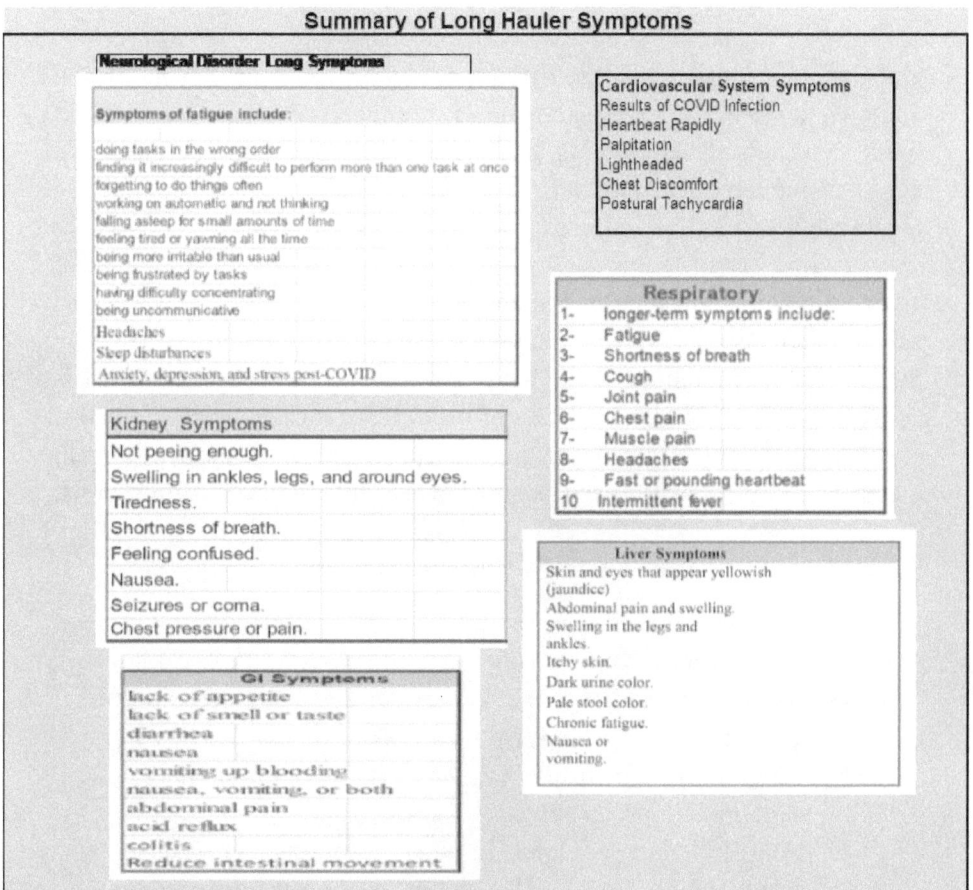

**Summary of Long Hauler Symptoms**

**Neurological Disorder Long Symptoms**

Symptoms of fatigue include:

doing tasks in the wrong order
finding it increasingly difficult to perform more than one task at once
forgetting to do things often
working on automatic and not thinking
falling asleep for small amounts of time
feeling tired or yawning all the time
being more irritable than usual
being frustrated by tasks
having difficulty concentrating
being uncommunicative
Headaches
Sleep disturbances
Anxiety, depression, and stress post-COVID

**Cardiovascular System Symptoms**
Results of COVID Infection
Heartbeat Rapidly
Palpitation
Lightheaded
Chest Discomfort
Postural Tachycardia

**Respiratory**
1- longer-term symptoms include:
2- Fatigue
3- Shortness of breath
4- Cough
5- Joint pain
6- Chest pain
7- Muscle pain
8- Headaches
9- Fast or pounding heartbeat
10 Intermittent fever

**Kidney Symptoms**
Not peeing enough.
Swelling in ankles, legs, and around eyes.
Tiredness.
Shortness of breath.
Feeling confused.
Nausea.
Seizures or coma.
Chest pressure or pain.

**Liver Symptoms**
Skin and eyes that appear yellowish (jaundice)
Abdominal pain and swelling.
Swelling in the legs and ankles.
Itchy skin.
Dark urine color.
Pale stool color.
Chronic fatigue.
Nausea or vomiting.

**GI Symptoms**
lack of appetite
lack of smell or taste
diarrhea
nausea
vomiting up blooding
nausea, vomiting, or both
abdominal pain
acid reflux
colitis
Reduce intestinal movement

# Section Nine Ras System

## 9.0 RAS System

Once renin has been released into the blood, it can act on its target, angiotensinogen. Angiotensinogen is produced in the liver and is found continuously circulating in the plasma. Renin then acts to cleave angiotensinogen into angiotensin I. Angiotensin I is physiologically inactive but acts as a precursor for angiotensin II.

The conversion of angiotensin I to angiotensin II is catalyzed by an enzyme called angiotensin converting enzyme (ACE). ACE is found primarily in the vascular endothelium of the lungs and kidneys. After angiotensin I is converted to angiotensin II, it has effects on the kidney, adrenal cortex, arterioles, and brain by binding to angiotensin II type I (AT) and type II (AT) receptors. The effects discussed below are a result of binding to AT receptors.

## 9.1 Angiotensin Trip Through Human Systems

A. Liver secrets Angiotensin
B. Renin secreted, by the kidney, cleaves angiotensinogen, produced by liver, to form Ang I, 2)
C. Ang I is converted to Ang II by pulmonary ACE zinc-metalloprotease.
D. Ang II binds to angiotensin type 1 receptors (AT1Rs) or it is transformed into Ang (1–7) by ACE2 zinc-metalloprotease
E. SARS-CoV-2 spikes of virions cells bind to ACE2, inducing ADAM17-mediated ACE2 shedding, which is possibly driven by spike N-terminal domain binding/recruitment of ADAM17 close to ACE2.
F. ADAM17-regulated shedding
G. ACE2 results in increased amount of soluble and active circulating ACE2 (sACE2).
H. **ACE2 can transform both Ang I and Ang II into Ang (1–9) and Ang (1–7), respectively.**

I. The excess of Ang 1–9 and Ang 1–7 signaling via the AT2Rs can induce hypotension, anti-inflammatory (IL-10), antithrombotic or prothrombotic pathway activation.

J. Advanced and untreatable stages of COVID-19 disease. The main and initial actors of the process are ACE2 and ADAM17 zinc-metalloproteases, which, initially triggered by SARS-CoV-2 spike proteins, work together in increasing circulating Ang 1-7 and Ang 1-9 peptides and downstream (Mas and Angiotensin type 2 receptors) pathways with anti-inflammatory, hypotensive and antithrombotic activities. During the late phase of severe COVID-19, compensatory secretion of renin and ACE enzymes are subsequently upregulated, leading to inflammation, hypertension, and thrombosis, which further sustain ACE2 and ADAM17 upregulation.

# Section Ten Human Organs Anatomy

This section contains collection of human organs anatomy for illustration purposes to assist reader understanding the organs part and COVID infection related to specific organs.

**Figure 1A: COVID 19 Structures**

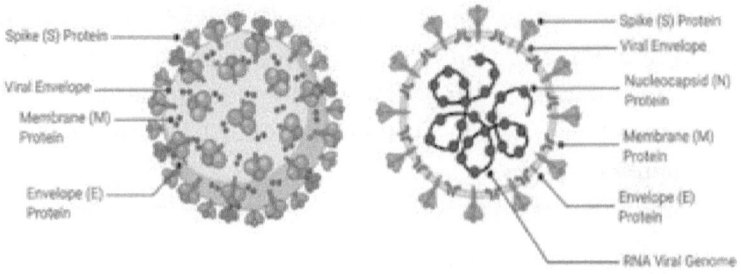

## COVID-19 Virus Structure

**Figure 2A:** OMICRON Showing Spikes Mutation

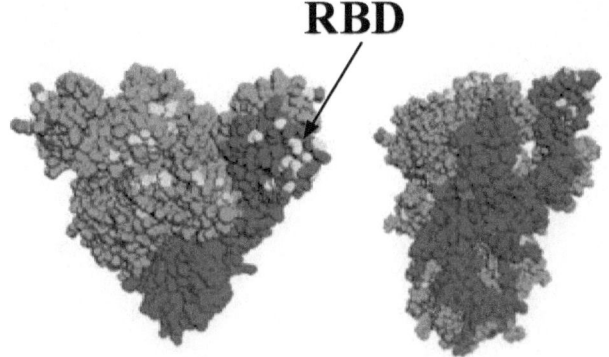

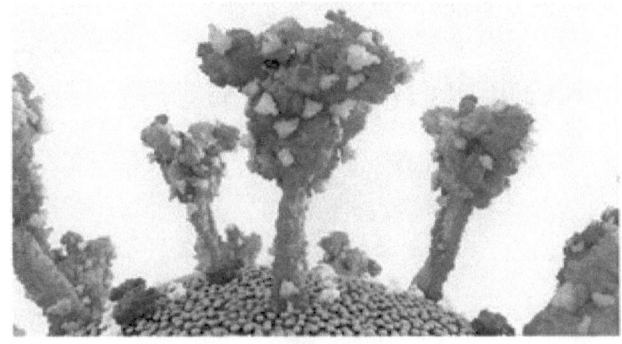 **RBD**

**Figure 3A**: Brain Main Parts

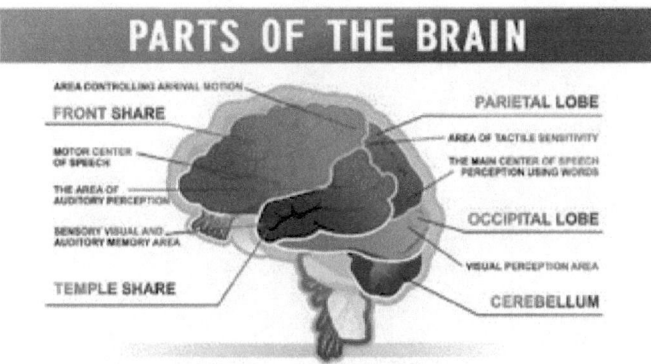

**Figure 4A:** Brain Main Sections

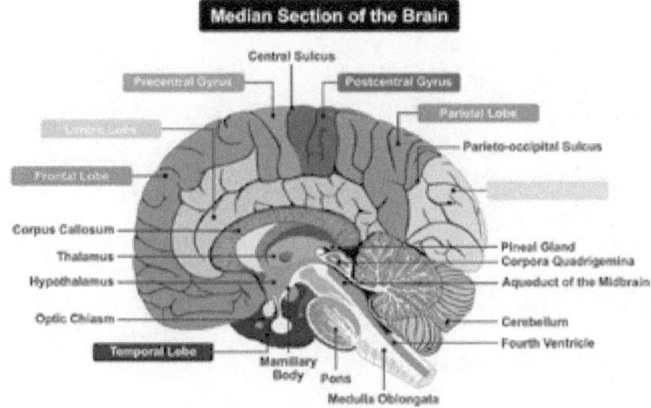

**Figure 5A:** Respiratory System

# Respiratory System

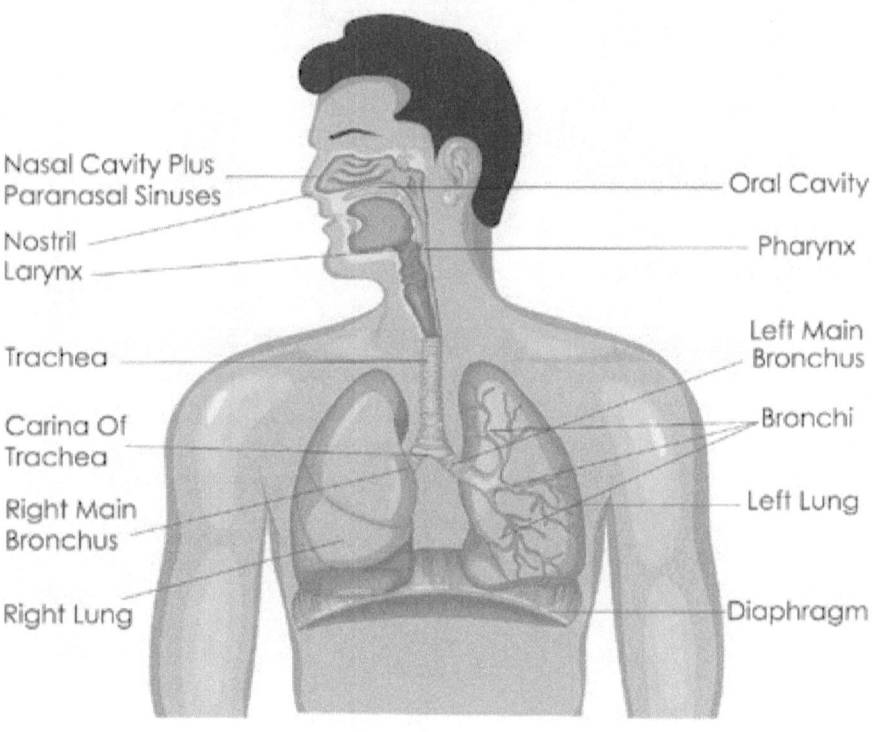

Nasal Cavity Plus Paranasal Sinuses

Nostril

Larynx

Trachea

Carina Of Trachea

Right Main Bronchus

Right Lung

Oral Cavity

Pharynx

Left Main Bronchus

Bronchi

Left Lung

Diaphragm

**Figure 6A**: Respiratory System in Details

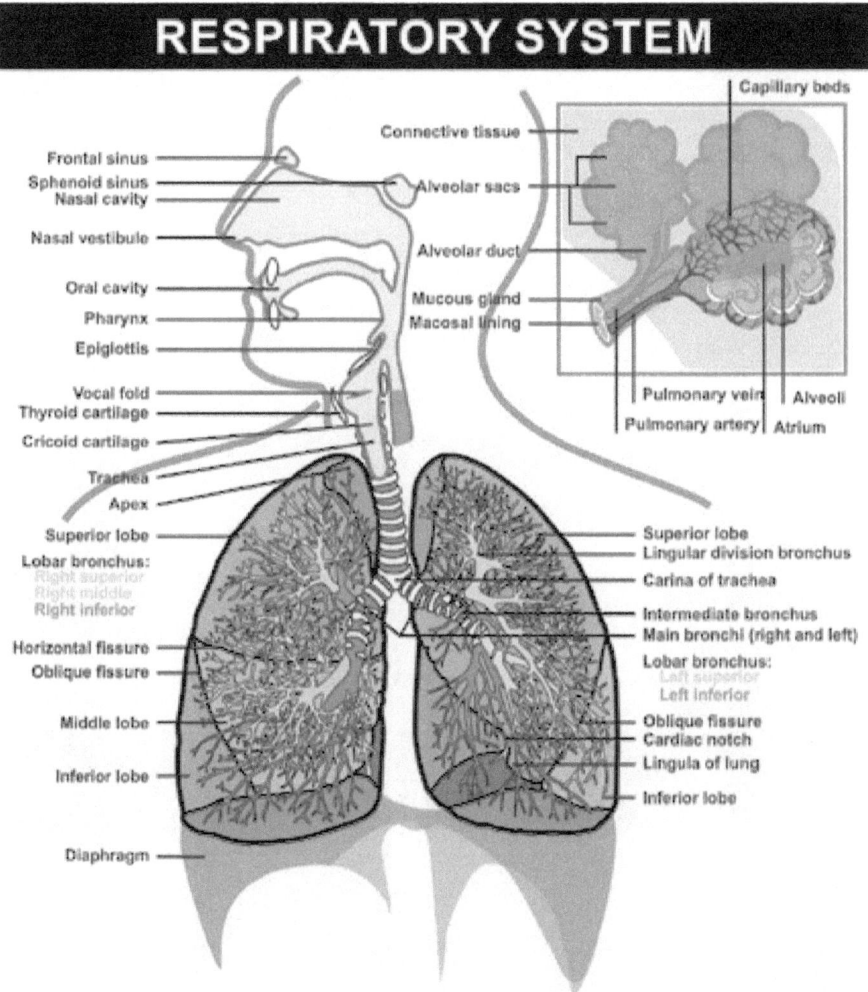

**Figure 7A:** Human Heart Detailed Parts

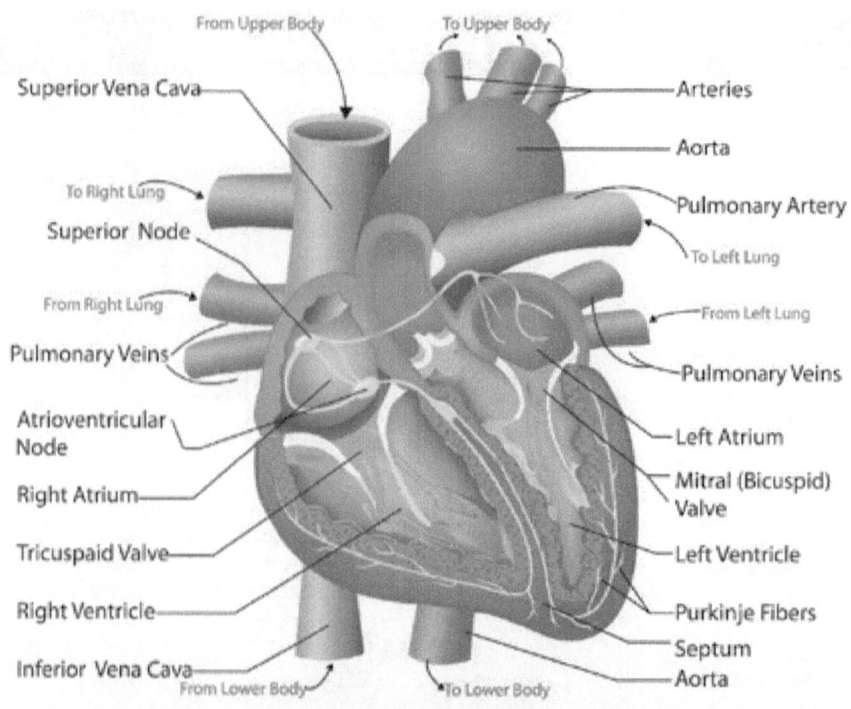

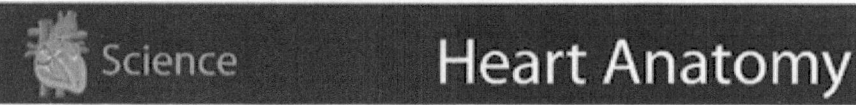

**Figure 8A:** Human Heart Blood Flow

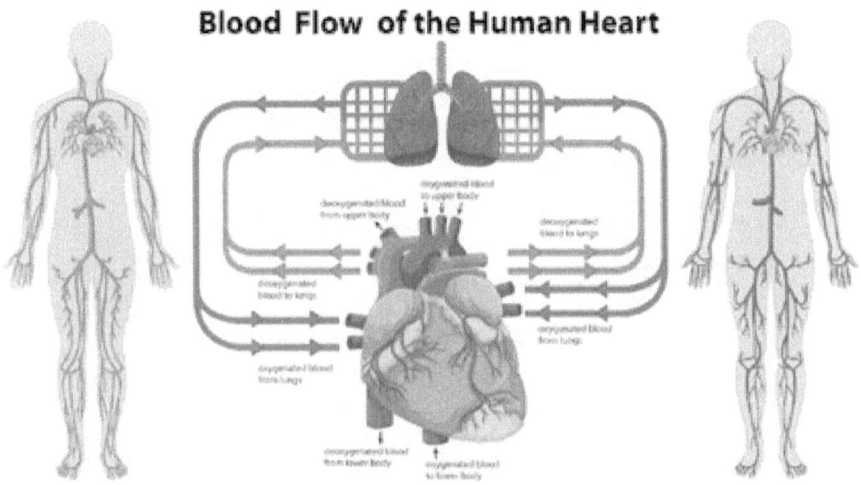

**Figure 9A:** Myocardial Infarct

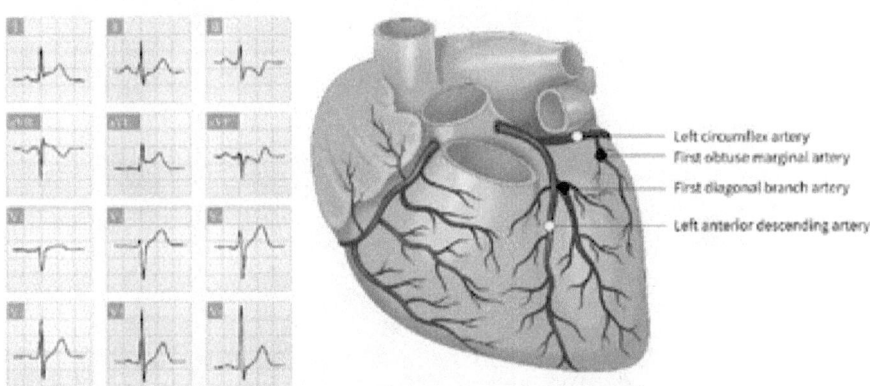

**Figure 10A**: Urinary System Main Parts

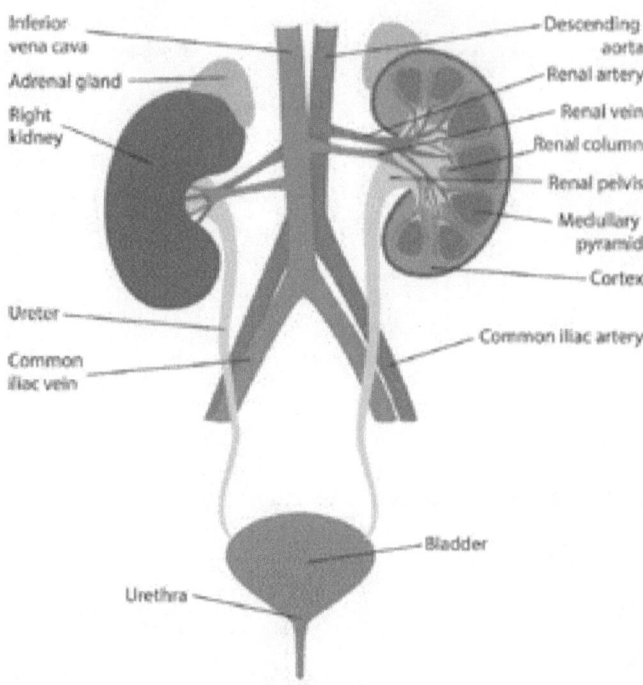

**Figure 11A:** Pancreas Anatomy

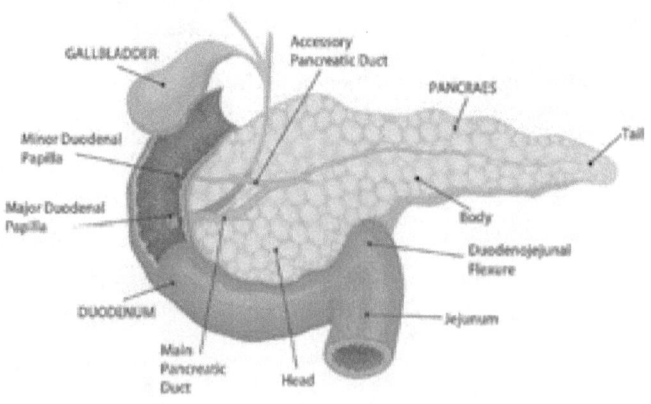

**Figure 12A:** Pancreas Islets

# ISLETS OF LANGERHANS

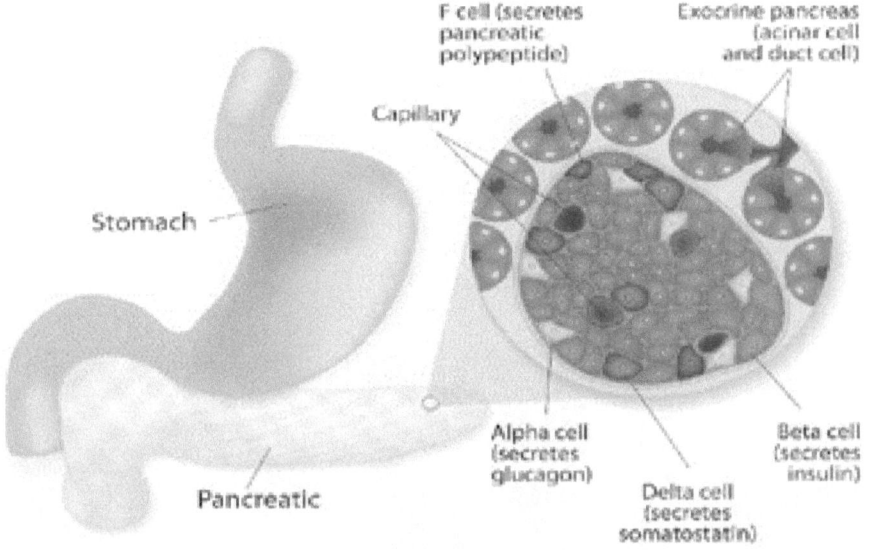

**Figure 13A:** Digestive System Functions

## Functions of the digestive organs

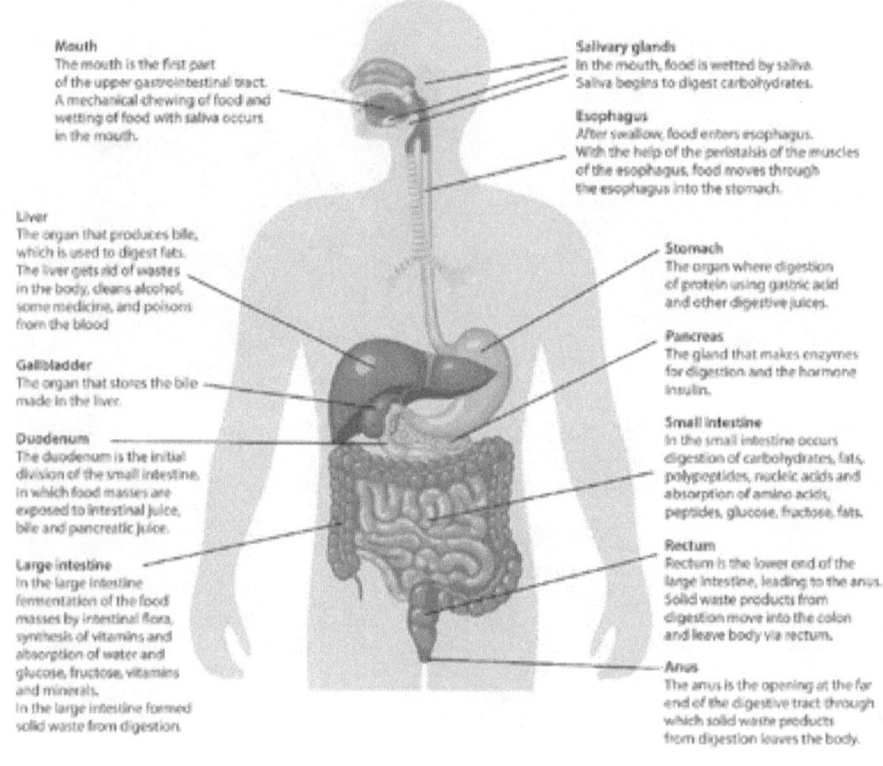

**Mouth**
The mouth is the first part of the upper gastrointestinal tract. A mechanical chewing of food and wetting of food with saliva occurs in the mouth.

**Liver**
The organ that produces bile, which is used to digest fats. The liver gets rid of wastes in the body, cleans alcohol, some medicine, and poisons from the blood

**Gallbladder**
The organ that stores the bile made in the liver.

**Duodenum**
The duodenum is the initial division of the small intestine. In which food masses are exposed to intestinal juice, bile and pancreatic juice.

**Large intestine**
In the large intestine fermentation of the food masses by intestinal flora, synthesis of vitamins and absorption of water and glucose, fructose, vitamins and minerals.
In the large intestine formed solid waste from digestion.

**Salivary glands**
In the mouth, food is wetted by saliva. Saliva begins to digest carbohydrates.

**Esophagus**
After swallow, food enters esophagus. With the help of the peristalsis of the muscles of the esophagus, food moves through the esophagus into the stomach.

**Stomach**
The organ where digestion of protein using gastric acid and other digestive juices.

**Pancreas**
The gland that makes enzymes for digestion and the hormone insulin.

**Small intestine**
In the small intestine occurs digestion of carbohydrates, fats, polypeptides, nucleic acids and absorption of amino acids, peptides, glucose, fructose, fats.

**Rectum**
Rectum is the lower end of the large intestine, leading to the anus. Solid waste products from digestion move into the colon and leave body via rectum.

**Anus**
The anus is the opening at the far end of the digestive tract through which solid waste products from digestion leaves the body.

**Figure 14A**: Human Lever

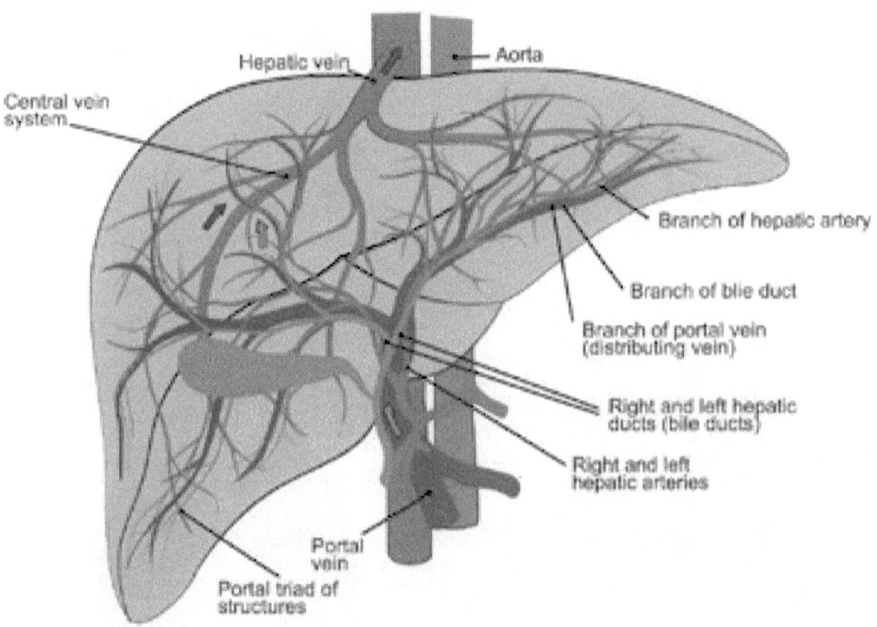

Internal Anatomy of Liver

Hepatic vein
Aorta
Central vein system
Branch of hepatic artery
Branch of blie duct
Branch of portal vein (distributing vein)
Right and left hepatic ducts (bile ducts)
Right and left hepatic arteries
Portal vein
Portal triad of structures

**Figure 15A:** Human Lungs

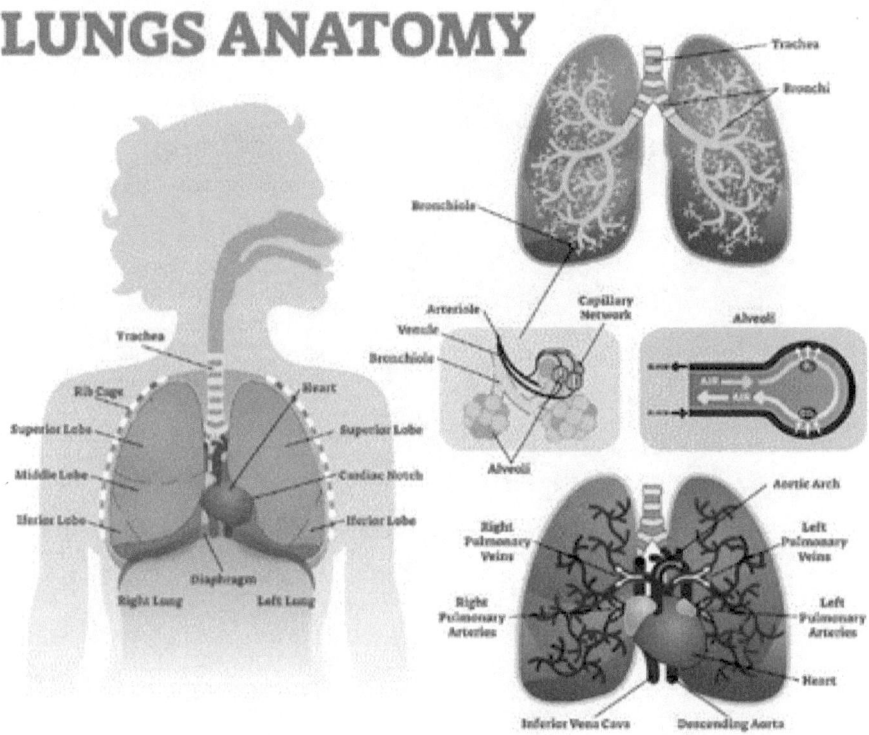

**Figure 16A**: Human Organs and Hormones Functions

# HORMONES

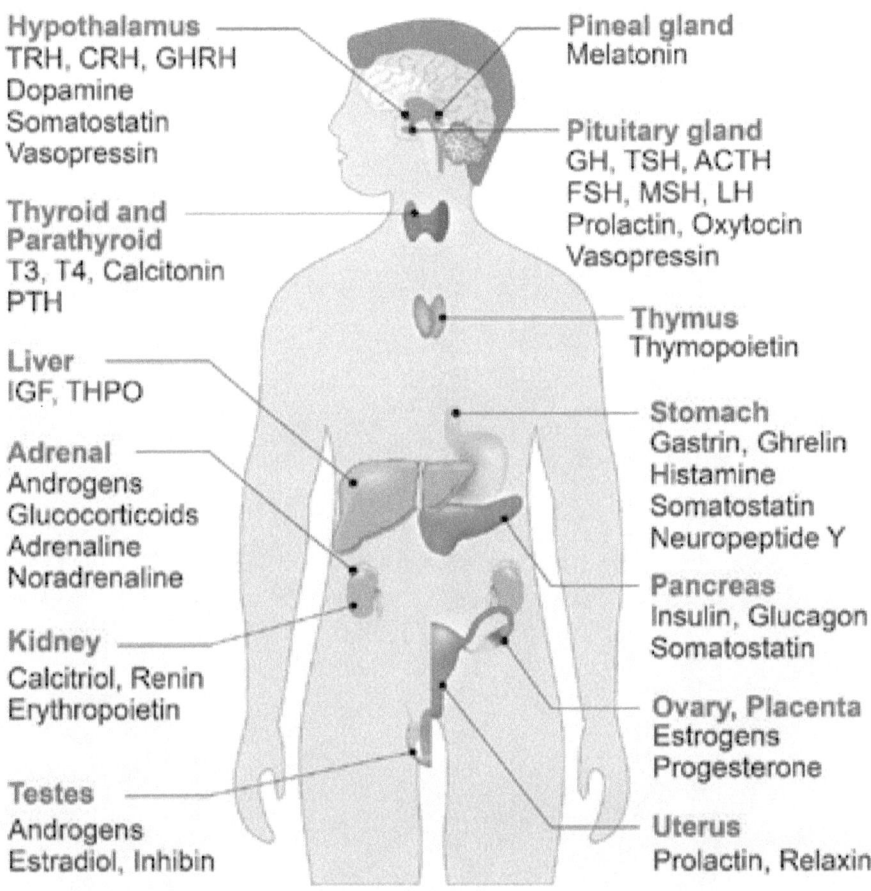

Hypothalamus
TRH, CRH, GHRH
Dopamine
Somatostatin
Vasopressin

Pineal gland
Melatonin

Pituitary gland
GH, TSH, ACTH
FSH, MSH, LH
Prolactin, Oxytocin
Vasopressin

Thyroid and
Parathyroid
T3, T4, Calcitonin
PTH

Thymus
Thymopoietin

Liver
IGF, THPO

Stomach
Gastrin, Ghrelin
Histamine
Somatostatin
Neuropeptide Y

Adrenal
Androgens
Glucocorticoids
Adrenaline
Noradrenaline

Pancreas
Insulin, Glucagon
Somatostatin

Kidney
Calcitriol, Renin
Erythropoietin

Ovary, Placenta
Estrogens
Progesterone

Testes
Androgens
Estradiol, Inhibin

Uterus
Prolactin, Relaxin